1,000,000 Books
are available to read at

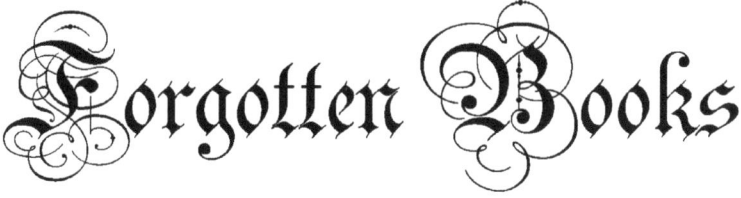

www.ForgottenBooks.com

Read online
Download PDF
Purchase in print

ISBN 978-0-259-20387-2
PIBN 10809569

This book is a reproduction of an important historical work. Forgotten Books uses state-of-the-art technology to digitally reconstruct the work, preserving the original format whilst repairing imperfections present in the aged copy. In rare cases, an imperfection in the original, such as a blemish or missing page, may be replicated in our edition. We do, however, repair the vast majority of imperfections successfully; any imperfections that remain are intentionally left to preserve the state of such historical works.

Forgotten Books is a registered trademark of FB &c Ltd.
Copyright © 2018 FB &c Ltd.
FB &c Ltd, Dalton House, 60 Windsor Avenue, London, SW19 2RR.
Company number 08720141. Registered in England and Wales.

For support please visit www.forgottenbooks.com

1 MONTH OF FREE READING

at

www.ForgottenBooks.com

By purchasing this book you are eligible for one month membership to ForgottenBooks.com, giving you unlimited access to our entire collection of over 1,000,000 titles via our web site and mobile apps.

To claim your free month visit:
www.forgottenbooks.com/free809569

* Offer is valid for 45 days from date of purchase. Terms and conditions apply.

English
Français
Deutsche
Italiano
Español
Português

www.forgottenbooks.com

Mythology Photography **Fiction** Fishing Christianity **Art** Cooking Essays Buddhism Freemasonry Medicine **Biology** Music **Ancient Egypt** Evolution Carpentry Physics Dance Geology **Mathematics** Fitness Shakespeare **Folklore** Yoga Marketing **Confidence** Immortality Biographies Poetry **Psychology** Witchcraft Electronics Chemistry History **Law** Accounting **Philosophy** Anthropology Alchemy Drama Quantum Mechanics Atheism Sexual Health **Ancient History Entrepreneurship** Languages Sport Paleontology Needlework Islam **Metaphysics** Investment Archaeology Parenting Statistics Criminology **Motivational**

SECRET REMEDIES,

WHAT THEY COST AND WHAT THEY CONTAIN.

BASED ON ANALYSES MADE FOR THE

BRITISH MEDICAL ASSOCIATION.

LONDON:
BRITISH MEDICAL ASSOCIATION,
429, STRAND, W.C.

1909.

THE LIBRARY
BRIGHAM YOUNG UNIVERSITY
PROVO, UTAH

TABLE OF CONTENTS.

	PAGE
CHAPTER I.—Catarrh and Cold Cures	1
„ II.—Cough Medicines	9
„ III.—Consumption Cures	20
„ IV.—Headache Powders	37
„ V.—Blood Purifiers	42
„ VI.—Remedies for Gout, Rheumatism and Neuralgia	50
„ VII.—Kidney Medicines	66
„ VIII.—Diabetes	76
„ IX.—Obesity Cures	83
„ X.—Skin Diseases	105
„ XI.—Medicines for Baldness	114
„ XII.—Cancer Remedies	117
„ XIII.—Remedies for Epilepsy	124
„ XIV.—Soothing, Teething and Cooling Powders for Infants	130
„ XV.—Remedies for Ear Disease and Deafness	134
„ XVI.— „ Eye Diseases	142
„ XVII.— „ Piles	147
„ XVIII.—Preparations for Rupture	158
„ XIX.—Cures for Inebriety	162
„ XX.—Cure Alls	170
APPENDIX	182
INDEX	185

A 2

PREFACE.

ONE of the reasons for the popularity of secret remedies is their secrecy. It is a case in which the old saying *Omne ignotum pro magnifico* applies. To begin with, there is for the average man or woman a certain fascination in secrecy. The quack takes advantage of this common foible of human nature to impress his customers. But secrecy has other uses in his trade; it enables him to make use of cheap new or old fashioned drugs, and to proclaim that his product possesses virtues beyond the ken of the mere doctor; his herbs have been culled in some remote prairie in America or among the mountains of Central Africa, the secret of their virtues having been confided to him by some venerable chief; or again he would have us believe that his drug has been discovered by chemical research of alchemical profundity, and is produced by processes so costly and elaborate that it can only be sold at a very high price.

The British Medical Association considered, therefore, that it would be useful if not instructive to make analyses of some of the secret remedies, the virtues of which are so boldly advertised, especially in popular monthly magazines and weekly newspapers, and in diaries and almanacks pushed under the front door or dropped over the area railings. The results are given in the following pages; they have been classified under various heads, according to the particular kind of disorder for the cure of which the preparation is more particularly vaunted. The claims in some instances are so comprehensive that it has not always been easy to assign the nostrum its proper place, and for a few it has been necessary to institute a chapter on Cure Alls.

An inquiry of the kind is, from the analytical point of view, tedious and often difficult; for though the analytical chemist can easily and quickly identify the nature of inorganic salts in a mixture or powder, and estimate their amount, most vegetable drugs which exert any appreciable effect on the body owe their power to the presence of an alkaloid or glucoside. The active principle of opium, for instance, is morphine; that of cinchona bark, quinine; that of belladonna, atropine, and so on, and the chemist can recognise any alkaloids present in a mixture or pill. It is otherwise, however, with vegetable extracts and colouring matters, for which pharmaceutical science has not yet been able in all cases to supply easily applicable and conclusive tests, because for the most part they contain no active principle and are used in pharmacy for their agreeable odour or bitter taste, as vanilla or sorrel are used in cookery. Of the accuracy of the analytical data published there can be no question; the investigation has been carried out with great care by a skilled analytical chemist, who has controlled his results in various ways, one being that in every doubtful case the formula obtained by analysis has been tested by making it up and comparing the appearance, taste, and physical properties of the imitative mixture with those of the secret preparation sold to the public.

The articles in this volume have not been confined to a mere dry statement of the results of analysis. Care has been taken to reproduce the claims and exuberant boasts of the vendors, and the contrast between them and the list of banal ingredients which follow must strike every reader. This juxtaposition of analytical facts and advertising fancies is instructive and sometimes entertaining, the fancy is so free and the fact so simple.

It must not be assumed that the concoctors of these mixtures and powders and ointments show any particular skill in the compounding of drugs. On the contrary, they appear curiously indifferent to taste and appearance, and perhaps count on the belief, common among the poorer classes at least, that the nastier a drug the more effective it is. There is, at any rate, the excuse for this belief that the effort to subdue the repugnance to the draught produces a glow of virtue which may perhaps have a certain stimulating effect on the mind; the patient having not only spent his money but suffered some discomfort, is anxious to justify his faith by assuming himself to be the better for the double sacrifice.

It is not, however, only the poorer classes of the community who have a weakness for secret remedies and the ministration of quacks; the well-to-do and the highly-placed will often, when not very ill, take a curious pleasure in experimenting with mysterious compounds. In them it is perhaps to be traced to a hankering to break safely with orthodoxy; they scrupulously obey the law and the Church and Mrs. Grundy, but will have their fling against medicine. Usually, however, people of these classes take to some system. It used to be electricity or hypnotism or some eccentricity of diet; nowadays it is more often Christian Science.

Judging from the relative number of secret remedies advertised for different complaints, it would seem that the most attractive fields for exploitation by the "patent" medicine man are afforded by those diseases which are widely prevalent, and sufficiently serious to cause considerable suffering and incapacity, inasmuch as such disorders lend themselves to sensational descriptions of the dire consequences which will follow if the one and only real and certain cure is not purchased.

The estimates of cost given throughout the volume refer only to the ingredients, the prices of the various drugs being those quoted in an ordinary wholesale drug list, and take no account of the cost of bottles, boxes, wrappings and packages, very often a much more serious source of expenditure. The stamp duty levied by the Inland Revenue under an old Act of Parliament must also be taken into consideration, but, ostensibly at least, it is paid by the purchaser, for the full price of a nostrum is usually 1s. 1½d. or 2s. 9d. and so on, the extra 1½d. or 3d. representing the value of the stamp. "Store prices" have, however, invaded this, like most other fields of enterprise.

CHAPTER I.

CATARRH AND COLD CURES.

THE analyses here given of some of the proprietary articles which the public are induced to buy for the cure of ordinary colds and catarrh furnish a good example of the absurdity of the barefaced pretensions in which nostrum-mongers indulge, for minor ailments are by no means neglected by the makers of nostrums; if the price to be obtained is somewhat lower than in the case of more serious disorders the cost price can be reduced in an equal or greater proportion. Alarming accounts, too, of the evils to be expected if resort be not had to the advertised articles are not wanting. Thus, in the advertisement of one of the articles described below, it is stated that catarrh "invariably creates biliousness, constipation, pleurisy, asthma, bronchitis, catarrhal fever, and consumption"; also that "it is estimated that over 20,000 people died in the United Kingdom last year of consumption caused by catarrh." The remedy put forward for this malignant disease is shown by analysis to consist of a solution of a pinch of common salt with a trace of carbolic acid, the actual cost of the quantity sold for a shilling being one-thirtieth part of a farthing. The probability that many people would regard a slight cold in the head as not requiring a resort to a "specialist in chronic disease in every form" such as the proprietor of this preparation, is turned to account by a disparaging reference to the medical profession. "Catarrh," we are told, "in its chronic form (and the complaints arising from it) is a malady which has not, up to the present time, received that attention and research from the medical faculty which it deserves. Most practitioners have given it merely a passing thought, or poohed at it as a mere cold which would soon pass off, and perhaps give some light tonic to tone up the stomach." Another of the " remedies " described well illustrates the way in which the public is deluded by such " specialists "; camphor, quinine and ipecacuanha are frequently employed as domestic remedies in the early stages of a cold in the head, and persons who believe in their usefulness can no doubt be induced to buy a " cold cure " which professes to contain them in combination with other drugs, presented in a form convenient and agreeable to be taken; but in the tablets which are represented as consisting of cascara, bromide, quinine, ipecacuanha, camphor and bryonia, analysis did not reveal any appreciable traces of cascara, bromide, quinine, ipecacuanha, or camphor. The principal ingredients actually present were cinchonine, an alkaloid found in the bark from which quinine is prepared but cheaper than quinine, and acetanilide, a chemical better known under the name antifebrin, both in very small doses.

Many proprietary medicines of varied kinds are recommended for colds among a host of other complaints for which they are stated to possess curative powers. Apart, however, from such inclusive recommendations, a considerable number are put forward expressly and primarily for cold and catarrh, and it is a selection of these which is here described.

Dr. LANE'S CATARRH CURE.

This is prepared and sold by a Company giving an address in London. The price is 1s. a bottle, containing 2½ fluid ounces.

Much printed matter is supplied with this preparation, and a few extracts are here given:

Catarrh, in its chronic form (and the complaints arising from it), is a malady which has not, up to the present time, received that attention and research from the medical faculty which it deserves. Most practitioners have given it merely a passing thought, or poohed at it as a mere cold which would soon pass off, and perhaps give some light tonic to tone up the stomach. And therein lies the fatal error, for Catarrh is a disease that cannot be trifled with, as millions can only too surely testify.

. . . to let any part or organ of the system become diseased breeds the seeds of a host of other complaints, as all the organs of the body are in sympathy with each other. The cause of this is easily explained in a case of Catarrh . . . It invariably creates Biliousness, Constipation, Pleurisy, Asthma, Bronchitis, Catarrhal Fever, and Consumption.

It is estimated that over 20,000 people died in the United Kingdom last year of Consumption caused by Catarrh.

The speciality of myself and Associate Physicians is chronic disease in every form. Our library was selected to this end, and the Herbal World explored for this purpose—the successful treatment of chronic disease.

We have never seen one out of five hundred of the patients whom we have cured. Most cases can be treated just as well at a distance as if we saw them in person; as our experience enables us to judge correctly from a written description the nature and extent of the disease under which the patient is labouring.

The preparation is described on the wrapper as:

The *Only Reliable* and Effective Preparation for the Permanent and *Radical Cure* of this most dangerous disease.

The directions on the label are:

For Catarrh.—Pour one-half tea-spoonful in the palm of the hand, close one nostril with the finger, and inhale the liquid through the open nostril with sufficient force to carry the spray down into the throat. Inhale another half tea-spoonful through the other nostril in the same way; it is not advisable to swallow the Catarrh Cure—however, it is perfectly harmless if you chance to do so. Use night and morning and in extreme cases three times a day.

Analysis showed the composition of the liquid to be:

Phenol (carbolic acid)	....	0·4 parts
Sodium chloride (common salt)	....	3·3 parts
Water to	....	100 fluid parts.

The traces of impurities usually present in common salt were also found.

The estimated cost of the ingredients in $2\frac{1}{2}$ fluid ounces is one-thirtieth of a farthing.

VAN VLECK'S CATARRH BALM.

This balm is supplied by an American Company having an address in London. The price charged is 4s. 6d. for a package containing $1\frac{1}{8}$ oz.

In an accompanying circular it is stated that:

This preparation is perfectly harmless, readily absorbed, and through its healing, soothing action affords immediate relief and quickly cures Catarrh of the Nose and Head, Catarrhal Deafness, Hay Fever, Cold in the Head, La Grippe, Tonsillitis, Sore Throat and all inflamed, irritated conditions of the nose and throat.

The "Balm" was an ointment, contained in a collapsible tube. The directions on the label are:

First clear your head out thoroughly by blowing your nose, then squeeze out from the tube a piece of Dr. Van Vleck's Catarrh Balm about the size of a pea, on the end of the finger, and rub it well up into each nostril, hold the other nostril and snuff it up until you can feel it all the way up through the air passages in your head. For severe Catarrh in the Head and Cold in the Head also rub thoroughly over the outside of the nose and across the forehead and on the sides of the head just below the temples. For Catarrhal Sore Throat and Tonsillitis rub thoroughly on the outside of the throat and swallow at bedtime a small piece about the size of a pea. Do not get it into the eyes. This preparation is perfectly harmless, readily absorbed, and through its healing, antiseptic, soothing action affords immediate relief.

The substance consisted of soft paraffin containing a small quantity of phenol and about 2 per cent. of a mixture of volatile oils. Oils of eucalyptus, pumilio pine, and yellow sandal wood were recognized, and the respective proportions of these were estimated by comparing mixtures of known composition with the original. The results obtained gave the following formula:

Phenol	0·6 parts
Sandal-wood oil	0·5 ,,
Oil of pumilio pine	0·7 ,,
,, eucalyptus	1·2 parts.
Soft paraffin to	100 ,,

The estimated cost of the ingredients for 1⅛ oz. is ½d.

DR. MACKENZIE'S "ONE DAY" COLD CURE.

This is supplied by a Company described as of London and New York. The price charged for a box containing 30 tablets is 1s. 1½d.

This preparation is described on the package as:

The Best Cure ! For the Worst Cold !
A Speedy Cure in all Cases of Cold, Influenza, Headache, and all Neuralgic Affections.
Nature's Remedy.

Dose.—One tablet to be swallowed with a little water every two hours until relieved.

As a preventive, one every four hours.

Not for Children.

The tablets were coated with sugar coloured with ferric oxide (so-called chocolate coating); after removal of the coating they had an average weight of 2 grains. Analysis showed them to have the following composition:

Cinchonidine sulphate	0·83 grain.
Acetanilide	0·71 ,,
Camphor	0·10 ,,
Talc	0·21 ,,
Water	0·15 ,,

The estimated cost of the ingredients for 30 tablets is 1¼d.

KEENE'S "ONE NIGHT" COLD CURE.

This also is supplied by a Company giving its address as New York and London. The price charged is 1s. 1½d. a box, containing 30 tablets.

This is recommended in the circular enclosed in the box in the following terms:

Keene's One Night Cold Cure will break up any cold overnight; or money refunded! Influenza cured in three days. Guarantee Label around every Box. If Keene's One Night Cold Cure fails to Cure your Cold, your money will be cheerfully returned on presentation of Guarantee Label.

Keene's One Night Cold Cure is in Tablet form and contains nothing injurious, being chiefly composed of Quinine, Cascara, Camphor, and other Ingredients adopted by the Leading Medical Authorities for Colds in the Head, Throat, and Lungs.

The " guarantee label " is worded as follows:

GUARANTEE.

If Keene's " One-Night " Cold Cure fails to effectually break up any ordinary cold, return this Guarantee with box to your Chemist and he will refund price paid.

Cascara—Bromide—Quinine—Ipecac—
Camphor—Bryonia—tablets. 7½d. per box.
The Keene Co.
Irving A. Keene, Treasurer.

The tablets were coated with sugar, coloured with ferric oxide (so-called chocolate coating). After removal of the coating they had an average weight of 2·07 grains. Analysis showed that they contained no bromide, no quinine, except the minute trace occurring as an impurity in the cinchonine found, and no camphor in sufficient quantity to be detected; there was no evidence of any extract or other preparation of cascara, and if any were present, the quantity did not exceed a small trace; the alkaloid found did not give the slightest indication of ipecacuanha alkaloid; extract of bryonia may have been present, as it has no distinctive characters serving for identification. The ingredients found were:

Cinchonine sulphate	0·21 grain (approx.)
Acetanilide	0·32 ,, ,,
Calcium carbonate	0·25 ,, ,,
Starch	0·34 ,, ,,
Extractive and excipient	0·87 ,, ,,

In one tablet.

The extractive and excipient possessed no characters indicating the substance from which it was derived; it contained a small proportion of alkali in organic combination, equivalent to 1·2 per cent. of dried sodium carbonate in the tablet, and the mineral constituents usually present in vegetable extracts. The estimated cost of the ingredients for 30 tablets is ¼d.

MUNYON'S CATARRH TABLETS AND SPECIAL CATARRH CURE.

These two preparations, which have been at one time or another very extensively advertised, are supplied by a Homœopathic Company. They are stated to be manufactured in U.S. of America. The price charged for the tablets is 1s. a package, containing 17 tablets.

This preparation is recommended in the circular which accompanies it in the following terms:

CATARRH POSITIVELY CURED.—Are you a sufferer with catarrh? Have you taken all sorts of drugs and patent nostrums? Are you tired of paying big doctor bills without being cured? Are you willing to spend two shillings for a cure that permanently cures catarrh by removing the cause of the disease? If so, ask your chemist for a shilling bottle of Munyon's Catarrh-Cure and a shilling bottle of Catarrh Tablets. The Catarrh-Cure will eradicate the disease from the system and the Tablets will cleanse and heal the afflicted parts and restore them to a natural and healthful condition.

On the package it is stated that:

When used in conjunction with the CATARRH CURE, they cure discharges from the head and throat, dryness, soreness and scabs in the nose, pains in the head, and all symptoms of Catarrh.

The directions are:

Dissolve one Tablet in 20 teaspoonfuls of warm water and use this solution for thorough cleansing of the nose and throat, night and morning. Inject through the nostrils with Munyon's Atomizer or by snuffing.

The tablets had an average weight of 6 grains. Analysis showed the composition to be:

Sodium bicarbonate	1·87 grains.
,, chloride	1·81 ,,
Borax, partly dehydrated	2·20 ,,
Phenol (carbolic acid)	trace.
Gum	0·12 grain.

in one tablet. The amount of borax was equivalent to 2·58 grains of the fully hydrated salt.

The estimated cost of the ingredients for 17 tablets is one-twentieth of a penny.

Besides the "Catarrh Cure" referred to in the above as intended for use with the tablets, there is a "Special Catarrh Cure" which costs 4s. a package containing 460 pilules.

On the package it is stated that:

It cures the most aggravated cases of hawking and spitting of mucus, stuffy or oppressed feeling in the head, dryness or scabs in the nose, gloomy, dull spirits, difficulty of breathing, dropping of mucus from the head into the throat, and liability to take cold easily.

The directions are:

Take four pellets every hour. Half quantity for children.

The average weight of the pilules was $\frac{1}{2}$ grain. On first opening the bottle containing them a slight smell of alcohol was noticeable, but the loss of weight on drying was only 0·08 per cent. No medicament of any kind could be detected, nor any substance but sugar; determination of the amount of the latter showed 100 per cent. to be present.

From the odour of alcohol observed it is not unlikely that the pilules had been "medicated" by treatment with some dilute tincture, but if so, the amount of medicament so imparted was infinitesimal.

The estimated cost of 460 pilules is one-tenth of a penny.

BIRLEY'S ANTI-CATARRH.

The price charged for this fluid, sold by a London Company, is 1s. 1½d. a bottle, containing nearly 3 fluid ounces.

The bottle was accompanied by four pages of printed matter headed "The Birley Monthly Report," in which the "Anti-Catarrh" was included in a "List and Prices of Dr. Birley's Compounds of Free (or Unoxidised) Phosphorus," and described as "Special Remedy for Catarrh and Influenza." The following extracts are from the same circular, under the heading "The Wonders of Phosphorus."

Free (or unoxidised) Phosphorus, whose chief seat or situation is in the brain, is one of the most important elements contained in our bodies. Without Free Phosphorus there can be no thought, and very probably no life. . . .

One thing is proved beyond doubt, that the degree of intellectual thought depends upon the amount of Free Phosphorus in the brain, and just as the Phosphorus is unduly wasted, so does the brain power weaken. . . .

Free Phosphorus, it is thus shown, must be the saving agent—no other means is possible. This one element must be replaced.

The directions are :

For an ordinary cold take one teaspoonful every two hours until better, then every third and fourth hour, and finally night and morning.

For severe attacks, commence by taking a dose every hour until better, then gradually increase the period between each dose as attack abates. For Children, give half doses.

Analysis showed the presence of :

Sugar (partly as "invert sugar")....	74 parts.
Tartaric acid....	1·15 parts.
Phosphoric acid	0·07 part.
Alcohol	trace.
Water to	100 fluid parts.

No free phosphorus could be detected, but the odour when the bottle was first opened suggested the presence of a trace. From the presence of a trace of alcohol it appears probable that an alcoholic solution of phosphorus had been added, and that the phosphoric acid had been formed by its oxidation. If the phosphorus found were in the free state each fluid drachm would contain about $\frac{1}{80}$ grain. The liquid was of a light straw colour, probably produced by addition of a trace of colouring matter.

The estimated cost of the ingredients for 3 fluid ounces is ½d.

CHAPTER II.

COUGH MEDICINES.

THERE are probably few, if any, ailments more frequently treated by the sufferer or his friends, without recourse to medical advice, than coughs and colds. The remedies employed in such domestic practice include preparations like "linseed tea" and others made at home, but these no doubt are supplemented in very many instances by some proprietary preparation, either one of those so largely advertised, or the speciality of some local compounder. It might be contended that here, if anywhere, is a legitimate field for the maker of nostrums, and it is therefore of some interest to ascertain what is being supplied in such nostrums. The particulars as to composition and claims made which are given below show that they well illustrate the evils which inevitably creep into the dealing in secret remedies, and the downward steps which lead to purely swindling nostrums. One of the articles now described bears on the label the unusual recommendation, "For serious cases seek medical aid"; this preparation is recommended as a "valuable aid" in various complaints, and the fact that it contains morphine is stated clearly on the label, but information is not given as to the amount of morphine present. Less modest claims are made for competing articles, until we eventually reach such statements as "all that is necessary is to take one dose of the lung tonic in warm water on retiring to rest, and the cold will have disappeared in the morning . . . cure is quite certain," and "If it fails no other medicine will ever succeed." Again, while the presence of morphine in one of the medicines is plainly declared, as we have stated, this is not so in other instances. In one of those in which on analysis morphine was found to be present the advertisement begins with a "guarantee" that the medicinal remedies contained in the lozenges cannot injure the most delicate constitution, and includes the statement that they may be safely administered to very young children; in another case the specific declaration is made that "the cough pills do not contain opium," which would certainly be regarded by most people as meaning that they do not contain the active principle of opium—morphine; and yet this was found to be present. The uncertainty as to what the composition of a secret medicine may be at any particular time is illustrated by another of the articles described, which has in past years been the subject of legal proceedings in the course of which the presence of morphine was proved, but which is now found not to contain any.

The number of advertised proprietary medicines for the cure of coughs is very large, and the number of those but little advertised and having principally a local sale is still larger; the latter, as a rule, have a good deal of resemblance to the advertised preparations. A selected few of the most widely advertised of this class have been examined.

The information which chemical analysis can give as to the composition of proprietary medicines is necessarily limited to the recognition of those ingredients which possess more or less definite chemical properties. The makers, of course, can make use of any one or more of a long series of vegetable extracts which very much resemble each other, and of various sweetening and flavouring materials sold for the purpose. In the case of many secret preparations analysis can afford complete and positive information as to their composition; but this is not so in every case, owing to many preparations commonly used in pharmacy being devoid of definite active principles that can be identified, and possessing no characters distinguishing them from others of the same class. Many such preparations are likely to be employed in cough mixtures; and, as these medicines usually contain a large proportion of treacle, honey, extract of liquorice, decoction of linseed, or some other old-fashioned complex preparations as basis, the identification of small proportions of many substances which are likely to be present becomes practically impossible. Many of the drugs in recognised use for coughs, such as senega, Virginian prune, etc., as well as domestic remedies like horehound and coltsfoot, are practically safe from certain identification by chemical analysis for such reasons, and in some of the preparations described below such substances may perhaps be present in addition to the ingredients named. The receipts given are not put forward as necessarily representing the whole of the ingredients in the articles in question, but they probably include all those which are of any importance or possess any known curative action.

The chief interest in the composition of such medicines, however, centres in the presence or absence of more potent remedies, such as preparations of opium, ipecacuanha, etc.; and here the analyst is on surer ground. The extraction of minute quantities of alkaloids from complex mixtures containing large quantities of saccharine and "extractive" matters is, however, a matter of much difficulty, and their identification is complicated by the great similarity in the behaviour of morphine and the alkaloids of ipecacuanha towards the various reagents used in their recognition. In this connection it may be pointed out that one or two of the nostrums here dealt with have been the subject of fairly frequent legal proceedings in consequence of their having been sold without proper observance of the poisons regulations, and the evidence given in such cases has shown wide differences in the results obtained by different analysts of high standing, both as to the quantity of morphine present, and even as to the fact of its presence or absence. In making the analyses here recorded, great pains have been taken to obtain accurate results, and they have been confirmed by the employment of alternative methods, etc.; but the results can only be given subject to the caution just expressed.

KAY'S LINSEED COMPOUND.

This compound is sold by an English provincial company in bottles, price, 9½d., 1s. 1½d., 2s. 9d., 4s. 6d., and 11s. per bottle; the 2s. 9d. size contained a little over 5½ fluid ounces.

This preparation is described on the label, wrapper, and in circulars, both as "Linseed Compound," which is given as the registered trade mark, and as "Kay's Compound Essence of Linseed, Aniseed, Senega, Squill, Tolu, etc." On the label it is also stated that it

contains a preparation of chloroform and morphine, and it is, therefore, labelled Poison. It is Demulcent, Expectorant, Tonic, and Soothing for Colds, Coughs, Asthma, Hoarseness, Difficulty of Breathing, Consumption, and Simple Ailments of the Chest, Throat, and Lungs.

In a pamphlet enclosed in the package, this preparation is recommended to be taken for Cold, Influenza, Sore Throat and Quinsey, Pulmonary Catarrh, Bronchitis, Asthma, Consumption of the Lungs, Whooping-Cough and Croup. In most of these, however, it is recommended as a "valuable aid" rather than a positive cure; other articles, such as ipecacuanha wine, muriate of ammonia, cod-liver oil, and chemical food, as well as "Kay's Linum Catharticum Pills," are also recommended; while under Bronchitis we read:

In an acute attack, *i.e.*, when the symptoms are inflammatory with much fever, etc., *the family doctor should at once be called in.*

The directions on the label are as follows:

Scale of Doses { To be modified according to the age or debility of the Patient.
For over 21 years, a teaspoonful in water, at bedtime.
 „   12 „   half a teaspoonful „   „
 „   6 „   15 drops   „   „
 „   4 „   10   „   „   „
 „   2 „   5   „   „   „
Half Doses may be taken three or four times a day.
It is not intended for Infants.
For serious cases seek medical aid.

Analysis showed that 100 parts by measure contained 1·07 parts of chloroform and 4·3 parts of alcohol, both by measure, and 67 parts of solids; about 48 parts of the latter consisted of sugar, partly in the form of invert sugar, and the remaining 19 parts consisted principally of the mucilage of decoction of linseed; oil of aniseed was present, and evidence was obtained of small quantities of preparations of tolu and squill. The ipecacuanha alkaloids extracted amounted to 0·007 per cent., and the morphine to 0·021 per cent. If the ipecacuanha were present in the form of wine of the official strength, this represents :

Ipecacuanha wine	42 minims.
Morphine	½ grain.
Chloroform	5 minims.

in each fluid ounce.

OWBRIDGE'S LUNG TONIC.

This is sold by another English provincial company, price, 1s. 1½d., 2s. 9d., 4s. 6d., and 11s. a bottle; the 2s. 9d. size contained a little over 6½ fluid ounces.

It is stated on the wrapper that this :

Cures Coughs, Colds, Asthma, Bronchitis, Influenza, and all Affections of the Chest, Throat, and Lungs.

Also,

This Preparation does not contain any Opium, Laudanum, or Morphine, therefore does not require a Poison Label.

A pamphlet was enclosed in the package, from which the following is an extract :

Having once contracted a cold, however slight, it is of the first importance to have it thoroughly and radically removed. To do this it is worse than useless to rely upon a few lozenges, or any of the simple expedients to which many have recourse. Avoid linseed poultices, which are excessively weakening, and highly calculated to make the patient liable to a second, and, perhaps, more severe cold than the first. - All that is necessary is to take one dose of the lung tonic in warm water on retiring to rest, and the cold will have disappeared in the morning. The lungs and bronchial tubes will be fortified and invigorated to an extraordinary degree. Should the cough not be quite removed by the first dose, continue according to directions. Cure is quite certain.

The directions on the label were :

Scale of Doses.

Above 14 years	one teaspoonful.
6 to 14 years	half a teaspoonful.
3 ,, 6 ,, ...	fifteen drops.
1 ,, 3 ,, ...	five to seven drops.
6 months to 1 year	three to five drops.

Not to be given to a child under Six Months old.

To be repeated 3 or 4 times a day, if necessary. The doses given during the day should be mixed with a little cold water, the one at bedtime in a tablespoonful of warm water.

Analysis showed that 100 parts by measure contained 0·3 part of chloroform and 2 parts of alcohol, both by measure, and 89 parts of solids; about 73 parts of the latter consisted of sugar, rather more than half of which was in the form of invert sugar; it is probable that this had been added in the form of honey, and that the remainder of the solids consisted largely of the non-saccharine portion of the honey. Oils of aniseed and peppermint were present, and evidence was obtained of a very small quantity of a preparation of capsicum. The alkaloids of ipecacuanha were found to the amount of 0·002 per cent.; if these were present in the form of wine of the official strength, this represents:

Ipecacuanha wine	15 minims.
Chloroform	2 ,,

in each fluid ounce.

POWELL'S BALSAM OF ANISEED.

This fluid, prepared by a London maker, is sold in bottles, price, 1s. 1½d., 2s. 3d., 4s. 6d., and 11s. per bottle; the 2s. 3d. size contained a little over 3 fluid ounces.

In a circular enclosed with the bottle it was stated that:

This old and invaluable Medicine has the extraordinary property of immediately relieving Coughs, Colds, Bronchitis, Hoarseness, Difficulty of Breathing, and Huskiness in the Throat. It operates by dissolving the congealed Phlegm, and thus promotes free expectoration. . . .

In Asthma, Chronic Cough, Influenza, Difficulty of Breathing, etc., no pen can describe the wonders that have been wrought by this deservedly popular preparation.

The directions for use were:

For a Grown Person a teaspoonful two or three times a day. For a child about 8 years old, 20 drops; and 12 years, 40 drops.

N.B.—Grown persons as well as children should take it in a little gruel or warm water; or saturate a lump of sugar with the above quantities is a pleasant way of taking it.

Analysis showed that 100 parts by measure contained 1·8 parts of benzoic acid, about 4·2 parts of extract of liquorice, and 2 parts of sugar, 40 parts by volume of alcohol, and enough oil of aniseed to give a strong aniseed flavour; a very small quantity of an aromatic resin, apparently benzoin, was also found, and 0·012 per cent. of alkaloid. This alkaloid resembled morphine in its behaviour to solvents, by which all the commoner alkaloids were excluded; but other tests showed that it was not morphine, and it is possible that it was a morphine derivative, such as dionine or peronine, but it was not found practicable to establish its exact identity owing to the smallness of the amount. Powell's Balsam of Aniseed has, in the past, been the subject of legal proceedings on several occasions, and evidence has been brought in those proceedings proving that it contained morphine; so that it would seem that its composition has been changed since then.

Dr. KILMER'S INDIAN COUGH CURE.

This preparation, stated to be made in U.S.A., is advertised from an address in London. The price is 1s. 1½d. a bottle, containing 3 fluid ounces.

It was stated on the outside of the package that:

This wonderful preparation contains no opium, morphine, chloral, or other hurtful drugs, and therefore does not dry up a cough. Every ingredient is from Vegetable products which grow within sight of almost every sufferer. It will not only help but cure the most Chronic and Complicated cases.

The directions were:

Dose: ½, 1, or 2 teaspoonfuls every ½, 1, 2, 3, or 4 hours as the case may require. Children—less according to age.

Analysis showed that 100 parts contained 63 parts of solids, of which practically the whole was sugar; there was also present about 2 per cent. of alcohol and about 0·5 per cent. of oil of pumilio pine, with rather less than 0·1 per cent. of a resinous substance agreeing well with the resins from compound tincture of benzoin; a small resinous deposit also remained adhering to the inside of the bottle. A trace of a bitter yellowish substance was present, which may have been the aloes contained in the compound tincture, but did not agree perfectly with it in character; the quantity was too minute for exact identification. No alkaloid was present.

CROSBY'S BALSAMIC COUGH ELIXIR.

This elixir, sold from a provincial English town, and wholesale through a company in London, costs 1s. 1½d., 2s. 9d., and 4s. 6d. per bottle; the 2s. 9d. size contained nearly 4¾ ounces.

It was described on the label as:

A safe, speedy, and effectual remedy for Coughs, Colds, Hoarseness, Difficulty of Breathing, Wheezing and Irritation of the Throat, Hooping Cough, Asthma, and Incipient Consumption.

In circulars enclosed with the bottle, its use in these various complaints was more fully described; and it was stated further that:—

It contains no opiates, and is absolutely non-poisonous, and may therefore be taken with safety by the young and aged alike.

The directions given on the label were:

For Children, one month to one year, 5 to 10 drops in a little water. From one to five years, 10 to 20 drops. From five to ten years, 20 to 30 drops. From ten to fifteen years, 30 drops to one teaspoonful. From fifteen years and upwards, one teaspoonful, gradually increased to three teaspoonfuls, in a wineglassful of water.

Analysis showed that 100 parts by measure contained 65 parts of solid matter, about 58 parts of which consisted of invert sugar, 10·6 parts by volume of alcohol, a trace of chloroform, 1·35 parts of sulphuric acid, and 0·3 part of acetic acid; a trace of an aromatic substance probably derived from tolu was present, and a minute trace of alkaloid (much less than 0·001 per cent.); the remainder appeared to consist of extractive and colouring matter, and may have contained the non-saccharine portion of honey if the invert sugar were added in that form. A trace of acetic ether could be detected, and it is probable that the acetic acid found represented acetic ether originally added, which had undergone hydrolysis; in that case the amount of acetic ether originally present would be $2\frac{1}{4}$ minims in 1 fluid ounce. The sulphuric acid found corresponds to 44 minims of the official dilute sulphuric acid in 1 fluid ounce.

VENO'S LIGHTNING COUGH CURE.

This is prepared by a company in an English manufacturing town. The price charged is 1s. 1½d. a bottle, containing 2¾ fluid ounces.

On the label it was stated that:

If it fails no other medicine will ever succeed. It should be used in all cases of Coughs, Colds, Bronchitis, Pleurisy, Sore Throat, Hoarseness, Asthma, Croup, Whooping Cough, Influenza, and Catarrh.

In most cases it should be used with Veno's Lightning Fluid.]

Dose.—For an Adult, one teaspoonful; for a Child under ten, half teaspoonful; for an Infant, five or ten drops every two or three hours, during the day only.

Analysis showed that 100 parts by measure contained 7·6 parts of glycerine, 1·6 parts by volume of alcohol, a trace of chloroform, 0·23 part of a resin, 0·2 part of alkaline ash, and 1·1 parts of extractive and colouring matter. No alkaloid was present. The resin was not aromatic, and possessed no well-marked characters, but showed some resemblance to the resin of *Grindelia robusta*; the fluid extract of this drug is prepared with the aid of alkali, and the strongly alkaline nature of the ash found would agree with the presence of fluid extract of grindelia, but positive proof of the presence of the latter could not be obtained; the amount of resin found corresponds to about 7 minims of the fluid extract in 1 fluid ounce.

KEATING'S COUGH LOZENGES.

These lozenges are sold from an address in London in boxes, price, 1s. 1½d., 2s. 9d., 4s. 6d., and 11s. per box; the 1s. 1½d. size contained 50 lozenges.

A circular enclosed in the package was headed:

Notice—Guarantee.

The medicinal remedies contained in these lozenges cannot injure the most delicate constitution.

Another extract from the circular stated:

Very many also of the Nobility and Clergy, and of the public generally, use them *under the recommendation of some of the most eminent of the Faculty.* Such medical testimony must be convincing of their efficacy as well as conveying the satisfactory assurance of their freedom from any medicine, in the slightest degree injurious to the constitution, Medical Men being well aware of the deleterious effects of many preparations, which in Pulmonary Affections do but mask the symptoms for a time, and afford only temporary relief, while perhaps the constitutional disease is aggravated, or at least unsubdued. They may be safely administered to females of the most delicate frame, and to very young children, for they not only allay Cough and Nervous Irritation, but they sustain the constitution, by promoting a healthy state of the Digestive Organs. They have immediate influence over the following cases:—*Asthmatic and Consumptive Complaints, Coughs, Shortness of Breath, Hoarseness, etc., etc.*

Directions for Use. One or two, taken at bedtime, will allay the irritation in the Throat, and prevent the Cough from disturbing the patient during the night, *and one also eight or ten times in the day,* when the Cough is troublesome, will afford great relief.

The average weight of the lozenges was 16½ grains; analysis showed that they contained morphine, alkaloids of ipecacuanha, extract of liquorice, sugar (partly as invert sugar), and gum; some evidence was also obtained of the presence of extract of squill and tolu, but positive proof of the identity of these was not obtainable. The proportions of the various ingredients found corresponded to:

Morphine	0·007 grain.
Ipecacuanha	0·07 ,,
Extract of liquorice	2·1 grains.
Sugars	13 ,,

in one lozenge.

BEECHAM'S COUGH PILLS.

These cough pills, sold from a town in Lancashire, cost 1s. 1½d. per box, containing 56 pills.

The following extracts are from a circular enclosed with the box:

Persons suffering from Cough and kindred troubles should relieve their minds of the idea that nothing will benefit them unless it be in the form of a lozenge, or taken as liquid. Let them try *Beecham's Cough Pills*, and they will never regret it.

The *Cough Pills* do not contain opium; they do not constipate; they do not upset the stomach. On the first symptoms of a Cold or Chill, a timely dose of Beecham's Cough Pills will invariably ward off all dangerous features. For years many families have used no other Winter Medicine. Householders and travellers should avail themselves of this good, safe, and simple remedy for Coughs in general, Asthma, Bronchial Affections, Hoarseness, Shortness of Breath, Tightness and Oppression of the Chest, Wheezing, etc.

The doses may be from three to six pills morning, noon, and night.

The pills had an average weight of 1·4 grains. In spite of the statement that they "do not contain opium," analysis showed morphine to be present, together with powdered squill, powdered aniseed, extract of liquorice, and a resinous substance agreeing in character with the resin of ammoniacum. Approximate determination of the proportions of the ingredients is alone possible in such a mixture; the results obtained pointed to the following formula:

Morphine	0·0035 grain.
Powdered squill	0·1 ,,
Powdered aniseed	0·3 ,,
Ammoniacum	0·3 ,,
Extract of liquorice	0·4 ,,

in one pill.

SOME GERMAN NOSTRUMS.

Dr. F. Zernik, assistant in the Pharmaceutical Institute of the University of Berlin, undertook a short time ago, at the invitation of the Editor of the *Deutsche Medicinische Wochenschrift*, to report on some of the secret remedies which are thrown on the market in such numbers in Germany as well as England. It would appear that for the most part the remedies advertised in Germany are not the same as those most advertised in this country, but it is proposed in this and subsequent chapters to give some abstracts from the articles in which Dr. Zernik has from time to time reported the results of his examinations.

Dr. LAUSER'S COUGH DROPS.

Dr. Zernik found on analysis that these Cough Drops did not contain the ingredients alleged; there was for instance only 3·35 per cent. of alcohol, although the advertiser speaks of tinctures of 50 per cent. In addition to this small proportion of alcohol the mixture appeared to consist of a watery solution of liquorice, an infusion of senna root, some ammoniated solution of aniseed and small quantities of ammonium chloride.

REICHEL'S COUGH DROPS.

Reichel's Cough Drops cost 1 mark for a bottle containing 65 ccm., about 2¼ fluid ounces. The purchaser is supposed to take 15 or 20 drops on sugar or in water four or five times a day. It is an alcoholic fluid, smelling and tasting of arnica, pimpinella, and anise.

TUSSOTHYM.

Tussothym, in spite of the wonderful qualities claimed for it by the firm producing it, proved to be a weak alcoholic distillate of thyme, diluted with water but probably containing another indifferent drug. It is advertised as good for all diseases of the respiratory organs, and especially for whooping-cough.

Dr. B. ASSMANN'S WHOOPING COUGH REMEDY.

This Whooping Cough Remedy is, according to the vendor, so complicated that it is only made by himself, and cannot be obtained elsewhere. The packet contains forty powders, twenty of which are marked No. 1, and twenty No. 2. The chemical analysis showed that each powder, weighing 2 grams, consisted of milk sugar (lactose). No other constituent was detected.

CHAPTER III.

CONSUMPTION CURES.

NOSTRUMS and quack medicines vary greatly in the extent to which they constitute deliberate fraud. In the case of some of them, it is easy to believe that the makers themselves have a certain faith in their preparations, and recommend them in cases for which they are unsuited with that bona fides which arises from ignorance, assisted, unconsciously perhaps, by an appreciation of the profitable nature of the business. Such preparations frequently contain some one or more of the drugs in common use for the complaints for which the nostrum is offered, and are even, occasionally, combinations compounded in the first place from a medical prescription which may have been found useful in certain appropriate cases. The injury to the public in such instances arises from the excessive nature of the claims made, the excessive price usually charged, and the probability of the advertised medicine being taken in cases for which it is quite unsuitable, when it may do harm positively by its effects or negatively by preventing the sufferer from seeking proper advice.

But with other proprietary medicines it is quite clear that the makers cannot in the slightest degree believe in the claims they make; the " remedy " in these cases is some substance or mixture devoid of medicinal activity, or possessing some slight therapeutic property having no relation to the disease for which the nostrum is put forward as a cure. It is often, indeed, for inert preparations that the most extravagant and emphatic claims are made; the makers, and the advertisement-writers whom they employ, are untrammelled by any necessity of squaring their statements with the real properties of the thing to be recommended, and having set out consciously and deliberately to deceive, they are able to give their whole attention to telling the most effective stories in the most plausible manner, and reaping the maximum of payment for the minimum of expenditure. People who are ill or suffering are to be frightened with impressive pictures of the aggravated suffering and premature death that await them unless they take the "only cure" in question, therefore let them be frightened thoroughly. Careful suggestion will induce people who are not ill to believe that they or some of those dear to them are in the early stages of some disease; therefore let everything possible in the way of striking advertisements, personal letters, and repeated assertions be utilised to produce the result. It is the victim's money that is wanted; therefore let the price be fixed high, and the advertisements be written up to it. If it should be discovered by correspondence that so much cannot be cajoled or frightened out of an individual sufferer, the price can be reduced gradually as "special concessions," in return for which testimonials may be extracted.

Of quack medicines the sale of which is conducted more or less on these lines, two examples are described in this chapter, and other examples will be enumerated later.

One of the two now dealt with is "Tuberculozyne," largely advertised in Great Britain but apparently of American origin; it affords an instructive example of the methods of the Transatlantic nostrum monger. The two liquids sold under this name consist of little more than coloured, flavoured water, but the modest price demanded is £2 10s. for a month's supply. No effort is spared to induce the victim to continue the "treatment" month by month, in spite of the evident absence of any benefit, which is unblushingly accounted for by the seriousness of the particular case, while the necessity of getting the system thoroughly permeated with the remedy is insisted on. The sale of another preparation advertised as a cure for consumption, Stevens' Consumption Cure, is conducted in a very similar way, but this time the herbs are said to be African, and the odd names they bear certainly have a Kaffir flavour. The vendor considerately warns the public against American quacks and impostors and against the preposterous and wicked swindles of Polish or German Jews. Although Stevens is so engagingly candid about his rivals he follows the plan of sending one letter after another to any sufferer whose name he may have obtained, a system which seems to have been invented in America; it is certainly cheaper than bold advertisement in newspapers, and is apparently found even more satisfactory, as it enables the vendor to give individual attention to the depth of his correspondent's pocket if not to the severity of his disease. But Stevens has somewhat bettered his instruction, and his letters and circulars have a character of their own due to the effrontery of his attitude toward the medical profession. Persons who respond to the advertisement receive a list of questions to be answered by the doctor who has attended them, and are advised to continue under the observation of their medical man in order that the latter may be impressed by the marvellous effects of the remedy. Not long ago a circular letter was sent out to medical practitioners, asking them to treat consumptive cases "which defy all the ordinary remedies" with this secret preparation. The circular continues: "The great drawback to my cure, so far as the medical profession is concerned, has always been the fact that I would not reveal its formula. This is now done away with; its formula is 80 grains of umckaloabo root and $13\frac{1}{3}$ grains of chijitse to every ounce, prepared according to *British Pharmacopœia* methods." The farce of revealing a formula by the employment of such fancy names as these is one of the oldest dodges of the quack medicine man, and no such names as "umckaloabo" and "chijitse" appear in any available work of reference on pharmacy. Enquiries made in various parts of South Africa have been negative, experts in native matters being unable to ascertain that the names were known. Further, the Native Affairs Department of Cape Colony has caused enquiries to be made in the Transkeian territories into the question whether the native tribes there resident had any knowledge of " umckaloabo " and " chijitse," or of their reputed medicinal properties. The result of the inquiry was entirely negative. Nothing was known of any such plants, nor was it even possible to identify their names. Smith's *South African Materia Medica* contains no record of any such names as " umckaloabo " and " chijitse."

A similar system of repeated letters sent in series to the sufferer or his friends appears to be followed by the Weidhaas Hygienic Institute, Ltd., which carries on a home in the south of England but also treats patients by correspondence. The proprietors, who would seem to hail from Germany, issue a pamphlet with the title *Dum spiro spero*, which is made up mainly of the usual testimonials, but contains also a sort of outline of the physiology of various organs, taken from medical works. The pamphlet does not differ from the ordinary productions of advertising quacks; the terms are said to be very moderate, the more so as it is the rule to make one charge only for the whole treatment, the proprietors taking the risk of its being of long duration. It would seem, however, that this arrangement is not always followed, for in a " Diet Table " headed " Direction for Weidhaas Home Treatment " we find the following :

It is absolutely necessary that all patients, while under my treatment, shall take the " Star Tonic " regularly.

On Rising.—Take one cup of " Star Tonic." (This must be always taken in sips only.)

For Breakfast.—Take the delicately flavoured Nutritive Salts Cocoa, boiled in milk (which, being specially prepared for invalids, on account of the great percentage of nutritive salts which no other cocoa contains, is most suitable in your case. . . .

Between Breakfast and Lunch take one or two tumblers of milk. If possible this should always be taken in the form of Kefyr, one of the easiest digestible nourishing and strengthening tonics. (Full particulars of this are enclosed herewith.) . . .

Half an hour before mid-day meal.—(From 1 to 2 o'clock.) Sip one cup of Star Tonic.

For Mid-day Meal.—*Make it a strict rule to take regularly green vegetables of some kind, such as spinach, cabbage, lettuce, etc. A fair amount of these should be taken daily.* To these may be added a few potatoes, very little meat or fish, and now and then, in the place of the latter, some pulses, such as lentils (German are best). . . .

At Tea Time.—If absolutely necessary, take a cup of weak ordinary tea or health coffee; better still, take a cup of Star Tonic, some *cold* toast. . . .

For Supper.—(Let this meal be not later than two-and-a-half, or, better still, three hours before going to bed.) Take either Cocoa or Kefyr. . . .

Before going to bed.—Always make a point of taking one glass of Kefyr or cup of Star Tonic.

When in bed always have some cold "Star Tonic" near at hand, and sip some when troubled with cough or acute symptoms.

At the bottom of the diet table is a notice to the following effect:

"The above specially recommended articles can be had from the Sales' Department of the Weidhaas Hygienic Institute, Ltd."

In the circular, referred to above as enclosed, Kefyr ferment is offered for sale.

In one case which was enquired into of a young man who had been induced to obtain the treatment, his mother wrote to the institute complaining that the treatment appeared to have done her son more harm than good. The reply, after insisting that the remedy supplied was the very best cure for his complaint, continued: "As to it lowering his vitality, let me say that it is not unusual for patients to feel apparently worse in the beginning, but it only shows that the treatment is disturbing the cause of the trouble. Now, this is just what I want it to do. I want to disturb it and thus drive it out of the system. I hope then you will allow your son to proceed under my directions. Give the treatment a fair trial and it will do all that is claimed for it." The patient was at the time in an advanced stage of pulmonary phthisis, and died of haemoptysis, of which he had had two previous attacks, seven weeks after the letter quoted above was written. A month after his death a letter was addressed to him by the director of the institute in the course of which it was stated that: "Many patients do not gain immediate relief, or even partial improvement during the early stages of the treatment, but Perseverance and a faithful adherence to all my instructions will invariably bring about the desired result."

Among the papers sent to an enquirer was a printed form which seems worthy of reproduction, since it illustrates a method of getting into touch with possible patients, which appears to be followed with variations by other companies that appeal to the sick:

R. B.

HAVE YOU FRIENDS WHO NEED OUR TREATMENT?

If you know of anyone whom you think might derive benefit from the use of our Home Treatment, you will do them and us a great favour by noting hereon their names, addresses, and the trouble you believe them to be afflicted with. Upon receipt of the names we will send them information concerning our method of treatment, but will not mention your name unless you desire it.

Name.	Address.	Ailment.
....	....	....
....	....	....
....	....	....
....	....	....
....	....	....
....	....	....

Please return to The Weidhaas Hygienic Institute.

Some time ago a firm of pharmaceutical chemists in a provincial town received a postcard from a company which offered 5s. for the name of any patient suffering from diabetes, pointing out that "it is money easily earned." The pharmaceutical chemists expressed indignation at the attempt to bribe them to commit a breach of confidence, but such a request might not be so regarded by a patient, more especially if the advertiser lays great stress upon his benevolent motives, and his anxiety to benefit as many persons as possible.

But although this letter-writing system with its paraphernalia of biographies of the discoverer, typewritten personal letters, free coupons and guarantee bonds is much in vogue, there are other nostrums advertised in the old-fashioned way and sold at the familiar price of 1s. 1½d. for a small bottle. Among these are some old preparations for coughs, for which more emphatic claims as remedies for consumption have been made of late years. The result of the analysis of two of these will first be given.

CONGREVE'S BALSAMIC ELIXIR.

This preparation, advertised from an address in London, is sold in bottles, price 1s. 1½d., 2s. 9d., 4s. 6d., 11s., and 22s. The 2s. 9d. bottle contained 1⅔ fluid ounces, the 4s. 6d. bottle contained 4 fluid ounces.

On the outer package was to be read:

Congreve's Balsamic Elixir. Has had a World-wide Reputation for 80 years as the Best Remedy for Consumption, also for Asthma, Chronic Bronchitis, Coughs, Colds, and Whooping-cough. Safe and Effective. Free from any poison.

The following extracts are from a circular enclosed with the bottle:

In the most obstinate attacks of Asthma, which have threatened speedy suffocation, when the sufferer, harassed by excessive coughing, has laboured dreadfully for breath, with an acuteness of agony not to be described, this Balsam has restored the patient to health, after the medical practitioner had abandoned the usual means in despair.

In Pulmonary Consumption, the best remedy is this Balsamic Elixir, as most unquestionable Testimonials prove. It has been successfully prescribed in Consumptive cases regarded as hopeless by the first physicians.

Correspondence. Advice by letter from time to time will be given to any patient whilst continuing Mr. Congreve's Treatment, provided that the 22s. or 11s. bottles of Elixir are *obtained direct from* [the address given by the vendor in his advertisements] during the period of correspondence.

The directions were:

For adults.—Take a teaspoonful, alone or mixed with honey or lump sugar, three or four times a day, as the urgency of the case requires. Children from 8 to 15 years may take two-thirds of a teaspoonful; from 5 to 8 years, half a teaspoonful; from 2 to 5 years, twenty drops; at six months, ten drops; younger infants from four to six drops.

The "elixir" was a bright red liquid; analysis showed it to contain 28·5 per cent. by volume of alcohol, and 2·6 per cent. of total solids; the latter consisted of resinous constituents (about 0·5 per cent.), sugar (about 1 per cent.), a little tannin, colouring matter (apparently cochineal), and extractive. Alkaloid was present only to the extent of a trace, under 0·001 per cent.; the extractive showed no characters by which its source could be determined; the resinous material was of an aromatic nature similar to the resins of benzoin, storax, tolu, or balsam of Peru, and appeared to be derived from a mixture of two or more of these. No other active ingredients were found to be present.

THE BROMPTON CONSUMPTION AND COUGH SPECIFIC.

The "Sole proprietor" gives an address in a part of London remote from Brompton, but it is perhaps hoped that the name may suggest some connection with the well-known Brompton Consumption Hospital. The price charged is 1s. 1½d., 2s. 9d., 4s. 6d., and 11s. per bottle; the 2s. 9d. bottle contained 3⅔ fluid ounces.

The origin of the preparation is thus described:

This Specific is prepared from the Prescription of an eminent Physician, who practised nearly forty years in Madeira, he was celebrated for his success in the treatment of Consumption and diseases of the Chest. Upon a visit to this country some years since, he gave the Prescription to a late Physician, who tried it upon five hundred out-patients; its effect was wonderful; it acted like magic upon their Coughs, and prevented that great waste of strength and flesh peculiar to this disease. It will save the lives of thousands and prevent Consumption, by administering it upon the first symptoms of Cough, which will be immediately cured by a few doses.

In a circular enclosed with the bottle it was stated:

A Cough is the forerunner of Consumption. In England alone 50,000 people die of it thus constituting one-fourth of the nation's death rate annually. It has destroyed more human beings than War, Pestilence, and Famine combined; it neither spares the old nor young, "and there is no family in which this rapacious destroyer of the human race has not had its victim." It is a well-known fact that people with diseased lungs can live for years, and follow their usual avocations in life, provided they are relieved of the principal feature of the disease—the Cough—which shakes and destroys the very elements of the blood, upon which life is supported. How very valuable and important to all, then, must a medicine be which will arrest and cure so fearful a malady!

The directions were:

Dose.—One teaspoonful three times a day and at bedtime. It may be repeated at night, or at any time when the Cough is troublesome.—Children over five years of age, one-third of a teaspoonful.

The following appeared on the outside wrapper:

In conformity with the Sale or Poisons Act, 1868, this preparation, containing a minute quantity of Laudanum and Chloroform, must be labelled Poison, but its composition remains unaltered.

The preparation was a syrupy liquid of pleasant odour and taste, resembling diluted treacle. Analysis showed it to contain in 100 fluid parts, 61·4 parts of total solids; of this, 35·5 parts were glucose and 9·9 parts cane sugar, and 2·6 parts ash, consisting principally of calcium sulphate. Chloroform, referred to on the wrapper, was not present in sufficient traces to be detected; alkaloid was present to the extent of 0·025 part in 100 fluid parts, of which 0·015 part appeared to consist of the alkaloids of ipecacuanha, and approximately 0·01 part was morphine. The difference between the sugars found and the total solids would be fully accounted for by the non-saccharine portion of treacle; extractive contained in the preparations of ipecacuanha and opium used would also be included in this. Small proportions of other drugs having no well-marked characters might possibly also be present; there was no evidence of any further ingredients, but in the presence of so large a proportion of treacle small quantities of indifferent substances it would not be possible to detect.

About 1 per cent. by volume of alcohol was present; assuming liquid extract of ipecacuanha and tincture of opium to have been the preparations of these drugs used, the formula is approximately:

Liquid extract of ipecacuanha	0·75 part.
Tincture of opium	1·3 parts.
Treacle	75 parts.
Water to	100 fluid parts.

Estimated cost of ingredients for $3\frac{2}{3}$ fluid ounces, $\frac{3}{4}$d.

STEVENS' CONSUMPTION CURE.

This is advertised as manufactured only by C. H. Stevens. The price is 5s. per bottle, containing $2\frac{1}{4}$ fluid ounces.

This preparation does not appear now to go under any other name than that of "Stevens' Consumption Cure"; as regards its past history, the following extract from *Truth* Cautionary List for 1908 is of interest:

Stevens, C. H.—The proprietor of a remedy for consumption which has been put on the market in South Africa and England under the name of Sacco, and later in South Africa as Lungsava, the recipe for which is stated to have been long in use amongst the Kaffirs and Zulus. In connection with the advertising of Sacco in England, an article which appeared in *Truth* was circulated in a mutilated form, omitting a condemnation of its sale as an absolute remedy for consumption. Stevens has acquired a number of testimonials from medical men, who must now regret their precipitate action. He is now in England on a new campaign.

The claims made for this preparation were put forward in printed circulars, and in letters, apparently printed in imitation of typewriting, sent at intervals to an applicant for particulars of the cure. Extracts from these are here given:

It has been admitted the world over that there is no remedy known to the Medical Fraternity to really cure Consumption, so it is preposterous to claim the ordinary drugs that are known to every Chemist even, to cure this disease, just because they are given a fancy name, and advertised by a Polish or a German Jew; it is not only preposterous but a wicked swindle.

There is no other treatment, drug, or medicine advertised in Great Britain to-day to cure Consumption, the ingredients of which are not known to every doctor and chemist in the world, and if you cannot obtain relief from these under the care of your own Medical Adviser, how can you be cured by using them on the advice of an American Quack.

Your own doctor will bear out what I say. Most of these American Impostors come to England after the U.S.A. Post Office Authorities have refused to convey their letters.

I do not say in my advertisements " Consumption can be cured," " Consumption is curable," or any such evasive remarks, but I say " *I will guarantee to cure you* if you are consumptive, or *return your money* in full," and that my terms are " No Cure, No Pay."

The African herbs which my Cure is prepared from have never been used by any white Doctor or Chemist before I introduced same to civilization a few years ago. These herbs are original and have defied our cleverest Analysts to discover the active principals they contain. . . . .

I only returned to England a few weeks ago to prove my Cure to the satisfaction of the British Government, having been absent for many years. . . . .

It does not matter whether a Doctor is attending patients or not whilst they are under my treatment, although I always prefer a Doctor to be in attendance to see the cure being effected because I particularly wish to convince the Medical fraternity of the genuineness of my cure.

From the first letter:

Usually two or three weeks' treatment is quite sufficient to make a substantial improvement, and a three months' course, in most cases, is sufficient to effect a cure.

From the second letter:

Let me send you a two weeks' treatment, which is more than sufficient to completely stop the progress of the disease.

From a later letter :

In spite of the mountains of prejudice to be overcome, I intend to prove that at last something has been discovered that will destroy the Tubercle Bacillus without being detrimental in any way to the human system ; in fact, besides destroying this germ, it is a strong tonic, and will invigorate a healthy body as well as bring back to its normal condition a Consumptive one. . . .

Now you must know that throughout the world our clever Scientists and most Prominent Specialists on Consumption have for ages past spent their lives trying to find something which will destroy the Tubercle Bacillus without injuring the human system. They have had everything at their command ; the most up-to-date Sanatoria, the cleverest Nurses, and the pick of climates, yet they have failed, though every drug and remedy known, including every ingredient contained in any proprietary medicine or cough mixture ever heard of has been exhaustively tested in every shape and form. My treatment differs in this one great respect, that none of the ingredients have ever been used before by any Chemist or Doctor, and are an entirely original discovery. . . . .

I will give any Doctor its formula who requests it, and will supply him free of charge with all the treatment he needs for experimental purposes, and you must see that I can gain nothing by doing all this unless my treatment positively cures Consumption, as I claim it to do.

On the back of the printed letter quoted above appeared the following :

GUARANTEE BONDS.

The following are specimens of my guarantee Bonds. No. 1, I give to any sufferer who is considered by his Doctor to have at least six months to live in the ordinary course of matters. Terms of No. 2 Bond have to be mutually arranged. I do not accept any money under this Bond until all the conditions are fulfilled.

No. 1 Guarantee Bond.

To Mr.

In consideration of you having paid me £2 12s. 6d. for a three months' course of my treatment for consumption, I hereby guarantee that your health has, at the end of the three months, considerably improved to the satisfaction of yourself and also of your Doctor (who must be a practitioner registered in the British Isles) under a penalty of refunding the whole of the amount paid, viz., £2 12s. 6d.

(Signed) C. H. Stevens.

Broadway, Wimbledon.

No. 2 Guarantee Bond.

I hereby guarantee that it will be impossible to find any trace of the Tubercle Bacillus in your system, and that you will be completely cured of Tuberculosis (consumption) to the satisfaction of your own Doctor and the Government Laboratory on or before , 19 .

The only condition being that the sum of £ , is paid to me when this guarantee is fulfilled.

(Signed) C. H. Stevens.

Broadway, Wimbledon.

These are "specimens" of guarantee Bonds. Another document, however, which appeared to be the guarantee bond actually given, differed in containing a clause by which the patient:

> hereby agrees to take same [*i.e.*, Stevens' Consumption Cure] according to the directions sent out with the medicine, for three calendar months from date hereof, and to follow as far as possible the advice given regarding habits of life, diet, etc., and to fill in the form on counterfoil attached, correctly.

The "form on counterfoil attached" contained a number of questions to be answered by the patient, and also a portion "to be filled in by a Medical Practitioner after the above has been filled in by the Patient," including such questions as:

> How long have you attended to this Patient?
> Do you consider this a mild, severe, or hopeless case?
> Do you consider this Patient has a fair chance of recovery providing Stevens' Consumption Cure is all it is claimed to be?

and on the back the following appeared:

> This Guarantee must not be given by a chemist or any one else until it is signed by a registered Medical Practitioner to the effect that he considers the Patient to have at least six calendar months to live.

Thus the appearance was maintained of guaranteeing benefit or cure, and refunding the money if the undertaking were not fulfilled; but the conditions to be complied with were such that it appears unlikely that Mr. Stevens is ever troubled with applications for return of money under one of his "Bonds."

A "detailed direction sheet" was supplied, from which the following is taken:

> One teaspoonful in a wineglass of water (as hot as can be conveniently taken for preference) one hour before breakfast and two hours after the last meal in the evening, unless the patient be in the habit of waking between 12 midnight and 3 a.m., in which case an extra dose may be taken then. After the first week's treatment half-an-hour before breakfast is quite sufficient.

It appears that the use of this wonderful substance is not limited to consumption cases.

> Stevens' Consumption Cure is a vegetable germicide, fatal to all disease germ growths, but acts as a strong tonic; is a blood purifier, stomach cleanser, and a nerve stimulator; one will readily understand that it must be all these to cure Consumption and build up a broken-down system entirely by itself. Stevens' Consumption Cure can safely be advantageously given wherever a germ disease exists or is suspected.

One of the most recent circulars sent out by Mr. Stevens is addressed to medical practitioners, asking them to use his remedy in severe cases of pulmonary tuberculosis which defy all the ordinary remedies, and professing to give the formula of the preparation, as follows :

> Its formula is 80 grains of Umckaloabo root and 13 and one-third grains of Chijitse to every ounce, prepared according to British Pharmacopœia methods.

The medicine was a clear red liquid, and analysis showed it to contain in 100 fluid parts, 21·3 fluid parts of alcohol, 1·8 parts of glycerine, and 4 parts of solid substance; this solid substance contained about 1 part of a tannin and 0·2 part of ash, the remainder being extractive. No alkaloid was present and no other active substance could be detected. The solid substance agreed in all respects with the solids of decoction of krameria, or a mixture of this decoction with a little tincture of kino. The formula thus appears to be approximately :

> Rectified spirit of wine .... 23·7 parts by measure.
> Glycerine .... 1·8 parts.
> Decoction of krameria (1 in 3) to 100 parts by measure.

or it may be made with tincture of krameria.

Estimated cost of ingredients for 2¼ fluid ounces, 1½d.

TUBERCULOZYNE.

The Derk P. Yonkerman Company, Ltd., an American company with an agency in London, charges £2 10s. 0d. for a month's treatment and supplies two bottles, labelled respectively No. 1 and No. 2 Tuberculozyne, and containing in each between 11 and 12 fluid ounces of liquid.

The advertisement offered a book on "Consumption and how it may be quickly cured," and a trial of the cure itself, to be sent free. Application for the book and sample brought bottles of "No. 1 Tuberculozyne" and "No. 2 Tuberculozyne," holding about ½ ounce each, and a book of 48 pages dealing with the remedy. A few extracts from the book will sufficiently indicate the nature of its contents.

> There have been found cures for small-pox, and safe precautions, such as vaccination, prevent the spread of the disease; the horror of yellow fever has been dispelled by a remedy that amounts practically to a cure, and one could

always flee to a northern clime and escape it. The dread diphtheria also has yielded up its dark secret, and now is no more a stalking spectre; while yet dangerous it can be handled.

But through all these discoveries, consumption remained as mysterious and deadly as ever. It invaded the homes of the rich and the poor. It hunted out its victims among the inhabitants of the far northland of ice and snow, and it was just as persistent in the temperate zone and at the equator.

Climate, temper, condition of health or purse made no difference. One day the health and strength of the athlete, and the next day the fever of the consumptive; in a short time the frail skeleton would be laid away—another victim. That was the oft-repeated story of the " great white plague."

But this horrible, awful consumption, that has gone stalking through the land, should never again strike the same terror to the souls of brave men and women, and fill our hearts with such a helpless despair—for consumption can now be cured. Tuberculozyne (Yonkerman), the most wonderful and marvellous medical discovery of the age, cures consumption. . . . .

After researches lasting for nearly twenty years, the persistent efforts of Dr. Derk P. Yonkerman have been crowned with success, for his Tuberculozyne treatment has already been proved in hundreds of cases to be a specific of almost miraculous curative power. Its healing virtues have been demonstrated in not only the early stages of consumption, but in far advanced and seemingly hopeless cases as well. . . . .

Tuberculozyne (Yonkerman) was such a marvellous remedy that when its discoverer first announced he could cure consumption there were few ready to believe. He had, however, discovered certain salts of copper of remarkable therapeutic value, and his production was immediately subjected to the most elaborate and rigid demonstrative tests. . . . .

The consumption germs (tubercle bacilli) cannot live in the presence of copper, and as the Tuberculozyne treatment introduces copper into the blood, the consumption germs cannot live. . . . .

Intra-Venous Injection, after thorough tests under the most favourable conditions, proved absolutely ineffective. Trachael (sic) Injection has also been tried with equally unsatisfactory results. Inoculation with lymph from tuberculous animals not only utterly failed, but frequently hastened the patient's death. Antimony, prussic acid, emetics, blisters, mercury, iron, digitalis, clover, and numerous other drugs, have all proved useless, for they failed to have any action upon the cause of the disease, and only gave the patient temporary relief, if they produced any beneficial effects at all.

In treating consumption in the past, physicians making Tuberculosis a speciality have been accustomed to recommend creosote and its product guaiacol, while later arsenic has found a certain amount of favour. These physicians have undoubtedly been honest and conscientious in prescribing such treatment, for they were upheld by the practice of years, and the indorsement of the greatest specialists in each generation for a hundred years. Yet they were wrong; just as wrong and just as ignorant of the true remedy for consumption as the ancients were of geography before the new world was discovered.

Against the use of creosote or guaiacol, Dr. Yonkerman speaks positively and emphatically, and his opinions have now the support of all present-day physicians making Tuberculosis their special study.

A "Life History of Dr. Derk P. Yonkerman" was also given, from which it appeared that the home of Tuberculozyne is in Michigan, U.S.A.

The book was accompanied by a long letter, and this was followed at intervals by others; these were all printed to appear as typewritten, and dealt chiefly with the terrors of consumption if neglected, the importance of taking Tuberculozyne at once, and, after a supply had been sent, with the necessity of continuing its use even if no apparent benefit results. A few extracts are here given:

You need not be discouraged or believe your case incurable, even if you have tried all the usual remedies and found no relief, for hundreds of our cured patients have had the same experience; after all other remedies had failed to even stop the progress of their disease, they tried Tuberculozyne and were quickly cured.

From the third letter:

We realize that since you were taken ill your expenses must have been burdensome, and if you feel that at the moment the cost of a complete treatment of Tuberculozyne is more than you can readily meet, we will send you the full month's supply upon receipt of but 40s.; the remaining 10s. you may pay at your own convenience when you are fully satisfied that your cure is complete and permanent.

From the fifth:

It is therefore with a genuine desire to help you that we write enclosing a Special Voucher Coupon issued in your name, which will help you materially if the cost of our remarkable specific has been more than you could really meet. . . . This Special Voucher Coupon which we have issued to you is good for £1 Sterling when sent with your order for Tuberculozyne. You have only to post the coupon together with 30s., and immediately we will forward to you the complete treatment and full instructions for its use.

From later letters:

Even if her improvement is not at once pronounced, do not be discouraged; for in some cases the patients at first even seemed to be losing ground, but they persevered and finally were cured. It would be much better to take the treatment a few weeks too long than to stop too soon. . . . .

Just at this time, when the patient has been taking our treatment for some weeks and it is beginning to permeate her system through and through, courage is needed, for great improvement may not yet be apparent though her cure be assured.

Every letter was accompanied with one lithographed copy, or more, of testimonials.

The directions were:

After each meal, put thirty drops of the medicine from each bottle into a tumbler of milk; stir well and drink immediately.

If milk is distasteful, the medicine may be taken in water which has been boiled.

For patients between the ages of seven and fifteen years, give one-half of the above dose; for those under seven years, give five (5) drops only, from each bottle.

No. 1 was a bright red liquid; analysis showed it to contain in 100 fluid parts, 3·4 parts of potassium bromide, 12 parts of glycerine, a trace of a pungent substance, sufficient oil of cinnamon (or oil of cassia) to give a flavour, a very small quantity of alcohol, and cochineal colouring matter darkened with a trace of alkali; no copper was present. The following formula gave an exactly similar liquid:

Potassium bromide	3·4 parts.
Glycerine	12·0 ,,
Oil of cassia	0·1 part.
Tincture of capsicum	0·17 ,,
Cochineal colouring	q.s.
Caustic soda	0·06 part.
Water to	100 fluid parts.

No. 2 was a brown liquid, one specimen being bright and another containing a little sediment. Analysis showed it to contain in 100 fluid parts, 18 parts of glycerine, sufficient essential oil of almonds to give a flavour, and a colouring matter which appeared to be burnt sugar. No copper was found in the small free sample, but the larger bottle of No. 2 contained 0·01 per cent. of copper, and a trace of sulphate: this quantity of copper is equivalent to $\frac{1}{48}$ grain of crystallised copper sulphate in each fluid drachm. As regards the other ingredients the following formula gave an exactly similar liquid:

Glycerine	18 parts.
Essential oil of almond	0·1 part.
Burnt sugar	q.s.
Water to	100 fluid parts.

The estimated cost of ingredients for No. 1 and No. 2 together is 2½d.

The following notes on some German nostrums for Consumption are derived from Dr. Zernik's articles in the *Deutsche Medicinische Wochenschrift*.

KÖRBER'S CURE FOR CONSUMPTION.

The advertisements of this preparation are described as particularly flagrant. Treatment for a fortnight costs about 12s., and the medicine contains butter fat, honey, catechu and tar-water.

BACILLENTOD.

Bacillentod or "death to bacilli" also described as a "family tea," is advertised as a miraculous preparation which cures all diseases of the respiratory tract. In the prospectus the word "phthisis" is misspelt. One packet costs 1s., and consists of 85 grams of galeopsidis, the dog, flowering, or hemp nettle, a herb which is now quite obsolete but was an ingredient of "Lieber's tea for consumption," which used to have an extended sale,

HONEY COD LIVER OIL.

Pastor Felke's Honey Cod Liver Oil is recommended in preference to the ordinary forms of cod liver oil, on account of its pleasant taste and of the absence of any disturbing effect on the digestion. It is said to contain "fat extracted cod liver oil," whatever that may mean, but proved on examination to be nothing more than a mixture of 0·05 per cent. of cod liver oil with oil of peppermint and raspberry syrup.

CHAPTER IV

HEADACHE POWDERS.

HEADACHE is so common a disorder that it was to be expected that secret remedies asserted to be certain and safe cures would be extensively advertised, and the sale, especially to women, of headache powders, in most cases as proprietary articles, is at the present day undoubtedly enormous. Persons who may be disposed to resort to their use should, however, bear two facts in mind; the first is that headache is not a disease but a symptom, and that the only rational treatment is to ascertain and remove the cause, whether it be error in diet, want of exercise, local irritation of some nerve as by an unhealthy tooth, eyestrain, or some serious chronic nervous disease. The second is that fatal results have been known to follow self-treatment with antifebrin (acetanilide), which figures largely in most of them.

The powders analysed were in all cases obtained from ordinary dealers in unopened packages; the composition of each is given in such a way as to show the dose of each article in one powder of average weight. Since the separation of the ingredients depends largely on their different solubilities in various liquids, it is not possible to obtain quantitative results having quite the same degree of accuracy as in some other kinds of analytical work; but the results of analysis have been checked by preparing mixtures of the composition calculated and submitting them to the same analytical process; the possible error in the proportions given below does not in any instance exceed a very small fraction.

DAISY POWDERS.

The English Company which sells this remedy charges 7½d. for 10 powders; the average weight of one powder was 6 grains, but the weight of individual powders in a packet was found to vary from 5·7 to 6·4 grains.

The medicament consisted of acetanilide alone. Being an unmixed drug it was not liable to stamp duty, and the package was accordingly unstamped. The dose was stated to be one powder, repeated in two hours if necessary; half a powder for children of 12 years; not adapted for children under 12 years.

Two "certificates" were printed on each wrapper from individuals who are notorious for giving testimonials in the guise of certificates of analysis. The only fact certified was that the powders were "free from any injurious substance," in which medical opinion will scarcely support the writers.

The estimated cost of the drug (60 grains) in a packet is one-eighth of a penny.

The same Company also supplies "Head powders prepared by Daisy, Ltd.," the wrappers being printed in such a way that careful inspection was required to distinguish these from the powders sold as "Daisy powders." The "head powders" were found to consist of phenacetin only.

CURIC WAFERS.

These so-called wafers, also put up by an English Company, are recommended as a "safe and certain cure for headache, toothache, and neuralgia"; stated to be prepared "from the Prescription of an Eminent West-End Physician."

The "wafers" consisted of ordinary cachets, with the name of the article embossed on one face. They contained the medicaments in the form of powder. The package contained 12 wafers for 1s. 1½d. The average weight of the contents of one wafer was 8·2 grains, but that of the contents of individual wafers in a package varied from 7·3 to 9·3 grains. Analysis showed the composition of the powder to be:

Acetanilide	3·28 grains
Phenacetin	3·28 "
Caffeine citrate	1·64 "

Directions for taking the wafers were given, but it was not stated whether the dose is one or more.

The estimated cost of the drugs (98·4 grains) in a packet is nine-tenths of a penny.

STEARNS'S HEADACHE CURE.

This remedy, advertised by an American Company with agents in London, is recommended as "A Speedy, Certain, and Safe Cure for Headaches of all Origins, whether Sick, Bilious, Nervous, or Hysterical."

Like the foregoing it was put up in cachets described as wafers. The package contained 12 wafers for 1s. The average weight of the powder contained in one wafer was 9·8 grains; but the weight of individual wafers in a package varied from 9·3 to 10·2 grains.

Analysis showed the composition of the powder to be:

Acetanilide	3·92 grains.
Caffeine	0·98 grain.
Sugar of milk	4·90 grains.

The dose was one wafer. "If relief is not obtained, repeat in an hour; but more than two wafers should not be taken."

The estimated cost of the drugs (118 grains) in a packet is a little under ½d.

BELL'S FAIRY CURE.

This Fairy Cure, which is put up by an English Company, is stated to give relief instantly in all cases of neuralgia, headache, etc. A handbill enclosed in the package made further claims, from which the following extracts are taken, "guaranteed to be an instant and absolute cure" for "neuralgia, headache, brain fag, nerve pains." "Nothing else is like it. Nothing else is so good. Don't compare it with ordinary 'cures' or 'powders.' Fairy Cure stands absolutely alone."

Ten powders were sold for 7d. The average weight of a powder was 2·7 grains, but individual powders in a package varied from 2·0 to 3·7 grains.

Analysis showed the composition of the powder to be:

Acetanilide	1·16 grains.
Phenacetin	1·16 ,,
Caffeine	0·38 grain.

The directions were to take one powder, "repeat in an hour if necessary, then every two or three hours until a cure is effected." Yet it is guaranteed to be an instant cure! There was a notice that it was not to be given to children below 12 years of age.

In this case also an "analyst's report" was given on the wrapper; it stated that the powder "is composed of several organo-therapeutic agents well known in medicine"; probably the "analyst" did not mean quite what he said in the following: "In my opinion, the preparation is well calculated to fulfil the purpose for which it is intended, namely—neurotic affections."

The estimated cost of the drugs (27 grains) in a package is ¼d.

KAPUTINE.

This preparation, put up by an English Company, is stated to cure in ten minutes headache, neuralgia, and all nerve pains. In view of the similarity in composition of these articles, the claims to uniqueness are amusing. In this case the wrapper bore the words "Nothing as good. Nothing similar," while on the circular enclosed in the package it was stated that "Kaputine is composed of several approved ingredients. That is, unlike the white headache powders, which consist solely of one crude drug, and which have frequently been condemned as dangerous by the Medical Press—Kaputine is most carefully prepared from several ingredients which have the absolute confidence of the Medical Profession."

The price of 18 powders is 1s. 1½d. The average weight of one powder was 6·6 grains; the weight of individual powders in a package varied from 5·7 to 7·5 grains.

Analysis showed the composition of the powder to be:

Acetanilide	6·30 grains.
Ferric oxide	0·05 ,,
Sugar	0·21 ,,

That is, the acetanilide was tinted pink with what is practically the saccharated carbonate of iron of the *British Pharmacopœia*.

The dose was given as one powder: "If not completely cured in two hours, the dose may be repeated. Half a powder for children under 12."

The estimated cost of the drugs (119 grains) in a packet is just over ¼d.

HOFFMAN'S HARMLESS HEADACHE POWDERS.

These powders are prepared by a New York Drug Company, but the package also bears the name of another company, presumably the English agents. The powders are described as "a simple and effective cure for all headaches."

Ten powders were sold for 1s. 1½d. The average weight of one powder was 10·5 grains; nine out of ten weighed from 9·3 to 10·5 grains, the tenth weighing 15·3 grains.

Analysis showed the composition of the powder to be:

Acetanilide	5·02 grains
Cocoa	4·02 ,,
Sodium bicarbonate	1·01 ,,

The dose was given as one powder, to be repeated in half an hour if not relieved.

Estimated cost of drugs (105 grains), one-third of a penny.

WHOLESALE AND RETAIL SPECIALITIES.

In addition to the above proprietary articles, large numbers of headache powders are supplied singly by retailers, and are commonly bought for this purpose ready packed from a wholesale house. It was, therefore, thought worth while to examine a sample of such powders; the one taken for the purpose is known as the "Good as Gold" headache powder; three dozen were attached to a card for exhibition, and the powders are retailed at 1d. each. The average weight was found to be 2·8 grains, six individual powders ranging from 2·7 to 2·9 grains. The powders consisted of acetanilide only.

The estimated cost of the drug for three dozen powders is ¼d.

There is reason to believe that practically all the others sold in this way are of the same composition.

CHAPTER V.

BLOOD PURIFIERS.

ALTHOUGH, as a rule, the makers of any kind of quack medicine find no difficulty in showing that almost any disease that can be named takes its rise in the organs or part of the system which their own particular nostrum professes to benefit, it is, of course, particularly easy to connect a great variety of diseases with the condition of the blood. The claims made for some of the following "blood purifiers" do not fail in comprehensiveness, for ringworm and itch, among other complaints, appear to be regarded as disorders of the blood.

CLARKE'S WORLD-FAMED BLOOD MIXTURE.

This is advertised and sold by an English Drug Company, price 2s. 9d. a bottle, containing $8\frac{1}{4}$ fluid ounces.

The following passages are quoted from a pamphlet enclosed with the bottle:

No matter what the symptoms may be, the real cause of a large proportion of all diseases is bad blood. Clarke's World-famed Blood Mixture is not recommended to cure every disease; on the contrary, there are many that it will not cure; but it is a guaranteed cure for all blood diseases. . . . It never fails to cure Scrofula, Scurvy, Scrofulous Sores, Glandular Swellings and Sores, Cancerous Ulcers, Bad Legs, Secondary Symptoms, Syphilis, Piles, Rheumatism, Gout, Dropsy, Black-heads or Pimples on the Face, Sore Eyes, Eruptions of the Skin and Blood, and Skin Diseases of every description.

On the label it was stated:

The Mixture is pleasant to the taste, and warranted free from anything injurious to the most delicate constitution of either sex, which all Pills and most Medicines sold for the above diseases contain.

Directions: The mixture must be taken about half-an-hour after meals, in the following doses:—

For Adult Males.—One tablespoonful four times a day.
„ *Adult Females.*—One tablespoonful three times a day.
„ *Children under 12 years of age.*—Two teaspoonfuls three times a day.
„ *Under 12 years.*—From half to one teaspoonful, according to age, mixed with a little water and sugar.

Analysis showed the mixture to contain 1·5 per cent. of potassium iodide, 1·2 per cent. of sugar (partly inverted), 1·6 per cent. by volume of alcohol, and traces of chloroform and ammonia, a brown colour being given by a small quantity of what was evidently burnt sugar. The composition of 8 ounces is thus:

Potassium iodide	52·5 grains.
Spirit of sal volatile	10 minims.
Spirit of chloroform	67 „
Simple syrup	50 „
Burnt sugar	q.s.
Water to	8 fluid ounces.

The estimated cost of the ingredients is 1⅓d.

OLD Dr. JACOB TOWNSEND'S AMERICAN SARSAPARILLA.

This is sold by a Company having offices in London. A bottle, holding a little under 9 fluid ounces, costs 2s. 6d.

On the wrapper it was stated:

This Sarsaparilla is the great purifier of the blood and general juices of the system, it effects the most salutary changes in disease; cures scrofula, salt rheum, all scorbutic disorders, chronic sore eyes, rheumatism, piles, liver complaints, erysipelas, all blotches and eruptions of the skin; in short, it removes every impurity of the blood, and all humours and morbid collections of the body.

The directions given on the label were:

Take half a wineglassful three or four times a day, an hour before or after meals. Persons very weak and debilitated may begin with a tablespoonful and increase the dose as the patient recovers health and strength. It is better to take it without the addition of water.

Analysis showed 100 fluid parts of the liquid to contain 18·2 parts of solids, of which 5·5 parts were sugar (partly inverted) and 2·5 ash, the remainder being of the nature of a vegetable extract. The **mineral** constituents were only those common to the ash of most drugs, and no metallic salts were found in medicinal doses; nothing of alkaloidal nature was present. The mixture contained 8·1 per cent. by volume of alcohol. In the case of a vegetable preparation of this kind, containing no definite active principle that can be identified chemically, it is not possible to state with certainty the various drugs from which it may have been prepared; a study of its general properties, and a series of careful comparisons, pointed to the present mixture being of similar nature to the compound concentrated solution of sarsaparilla (liquor sarsae compositus concentratus) of the *British Pharmacopœia*, with the omission of the liquorice, and with the addition of sugar: the drugs in the official preparation (besides liquorice) are sarsaparilla, sassafras, guaiacum wood, and mezereon. A liquor prepared in this manner, with the alcohol reduced to the amount found in the mixture under examination and the aroma slightly increased by adding a little additional oil of sassafras, agreed fairly well both in general properties and the results of chemical examination with the medicine under consideration.

MUNYON'S BLOOD CURE.

Munyon's Homoeopathic Home Remedy Company has an office in London, but the label on the bottle bears the words "Manufactured in U.S. of America." On the outer package it was stated:

It eradicates all Impurities from the Blood, and cures Scrofulitic Eruptions, Rash on the Scalp, Scald Head, Itching and Burning, and any form of Unhealthy, Blotchy, Pimply, or Scaly Skin;

and similar claims were put forward on the label and in a circular enclosed with the bottle.

The bottle cost 1s. and contained about 200 pellets or pilules, of the average weight of $\frac{1}{2}$ grain. They consisted of sugar; careful search was made for small quantities of medicament, but no other ingredient could be detected. Quantitative determination of the sugar showed just 100 per cent.

The estimated cost of the pilules is one-thirtieth of a penny.

HARVEY'S BLOOD PILLS.

These pills are sold by a Company giving an address in Wales. A bottle, containing 20 pills, costs 1s. 1$\frac{1}{2}$d.

The label and the enclosed circular bear the picture of a man's head, with the words, "Harvey. Discoverer of the circulation of the blood," with the possible implication that the Harvey who discovered the circulation of the blood also discovered or invented these blood pills.

The modest claims made in the circular included the following:

Harvey's Blood Pills for Skin Diseases. An Unfailing Remedy for Scurvy Sores! Harvey's Blood Pills for Scrofulous Sores. A Certain Remedy for Ulcerated Legs! Harvey's Blood Pills for Sluggish Liver. The Surest Remedy for Ringworm! Harvey's Blood Pills for Erysipelas. The Quickest Remedy for Itch! Harvey's Blood Pills for Boils. An Effective Remedy for Eruptions! Harvey's Blood Pills for Rheumatism. The Safest Remedy for Piles!

Harvey's Blood Pills are purely Vegetable, and contain the best properties of Sarsaparilla, Dandelion, Burdock, and Quinine. They are Warranted Free from Mercury.

Harvey's Blood Pills fortify the feeble, restore the invalid to health, and do good in all cases. All sufferers should immediately have recourse to these celebrated Pills.

Harvey's Blood Pills are "specially" suitable for Females. They remove all impurities.

Somewhat lengthy directions were given for diet, etc., as well as for taking the pills, in various cases; from which it appeared that the usual dose is:

For a male adult, one Pill three times a day; a female adult, one Pill twice a day; children one Pill at bed-time.

The pills were coated with French chalk, coloured red externally; when deprived of their coating, the average weight was 2·76 grains. Analysis showed them to contain quinine equivalent to 17·3 per cent. of the crystalline sulphate, 21·7 per cent. of potassium iodide, small proportions of powdered rhubarb and liquorice, and vegetable extract or extracts. A mass prepared from the following formula agreed closely with the pills in general properties and in results on analysis in various ways:

Quinine sulphate	17 grains.
Potassium iodide	22 ,,
Powdered rhubarb	16 ,,
,, liquorice	8 ,,
Extract of sarsaparilla	12 ,,
,, burdock	12 ,,
,, taraxacum	12 ,,

Divided into 36 pills.

The estimated cost of the ingredients for 20 pills is ¾d.

PROFESSOR O. PHELPS BROWN'S BLOOD PURIFIER.

Professor O. Phelps Brown advertises in this country from an address in London; the bottle sold for 2s. 9d. contained 6 fluid ounces.

The following paragraph appeared on the label:

This medicine is a concentrated preparation of Rock Rose and Stillingia, combined with other plants, well known for their specified action on the blood, which makes a compound medicine, that has never been equalled, and will be hard to surpass in the scientific future. It is impossible to give a full account of its virtues and cleansing capacities on this label, and the Prof. must, therefore, be content with briefly stating that it is an infallible remedy for All Diseases of the Blood, be they Constitutional, Hereditary, or of Recent Contraction. Nearly every ailment known to the medical faculty is in a greater or lesser degree dependent for its appearance and its virulence upon a *Disease of the Blood*. Ulcers, Tumours, Scrofula Bunches, Fistula, Piles, Painful Eruptions, indeed all afflictions manifested upon the outer surface of the body are the consequences of diseased blood. Many terrible maladies, which take the shape of Internal Inflammation, Sores, etc., and appear in the form of Fevers, Aches, Swellings, Glandular Disturbances, Mental Derangement, and General Debility, also proceed from the same cause. It is an admitted fact that, with Pure Blood and Regular Bowels, no individual ever can be permanently, seriously, or dangerously ill, if ill at all.

Dose.—For Adults, one tablespoonful three times a day before eating. For Children, the dose must be reduced to a teaspoonful.

Analysis showed 100 fluid parts of the liquid to contain 19·7 parts of solids, of which 15·5 parts were sugar (partly inverted); a good deal of mucilage was present, but no alkaloid and no mineral substance except the small quantity of ash always present in vegetable extracts; alcohol was present to the extent of 23 per cent. by volume. Evidence was obtained of the *probable* presence of a preparation of stillingia, but this drug does not contain any active principle by which it can be certainly identified. Rock rose (*Cistus canadensis*) has been used to some slight extent medicinally, but no particular virtues appear to have been assigned to it; it is, however, described as bitter and astringent. The 3 or 4 per cent. of extractive matter present in the mixture under consideration showed neither bitterness nor astringency, nor any property by which it could be identified, or which would indicate any medicinal properties.

HOOD'S COMPOUND EXTRACT OF SARSAPARILLA.

This is an American preparation, but the Company which makes it has offices in London. A bottle, costing 1s. 1½d., contains 2¼ fluid ounces.

The following paragraph appeared on the covering of the bottle :

A trial bottle will convince the most skeptical of the real merit of Hood's Sarsaparilla, and will enable everybody to test its wonderful power in restoring and invigorating the whole system, in renovating and enriching the blood, in giving an appetite and a tone to the stomach, in eradicating and curing Scrofula, Scrofulous Humors, Scald Head, Syphilitic Affections, Cancerous Humors, Ringworms, Salt Rheum, Boils, Pimples and Humors on the Face, Catarrh, Headache, Dizziness, Faintness at the Stomach, Constipation, Pains in the Back, Female Weakness, General Debility, Costiveness, Biliousness, and all diseases arising from an impure state or low condition of the blood. Hood's Sarsaparilla is designed to act upon the blood, and through that upon all the organs and tissues of the body. It has a specific action also upon the *secretions* and *excretions*, and assists nature to expel from the system all humors, *impure particles and effete matter* through the lungs, the liver, the kidneys, and the skin. It effectually aids *weak, impaired, and debilitated organs*, invigorates the *nervous system*, tones and strengthens the *digestive organs*, and imparts new life and energy to all the functions of the body. The peculiar point of this medicine is that it strengthens and builds up the system while it eradicates disease.

In a pamphlet enclosed with the bottle it was stated :

It is carefully prepared from Sarsaparilla, Dandelion, Mandrake, Dock, Pipsissewa, Juniper Berries, and other valuable vegetable remedies, in such a peculiar manner as to retain the full curative value of each ingredient used.

The dose was given as :

Adult, $\frac{1}{2}$ to 2 teaspoonfuls; usual dose 1 teaspoonful three times a day; children, less, according to age.

Analysis showed it to contain, in 100 parts by measure, potassium iodide 1·7 parts ($7\frac{1}{2}$ grains in 1 fluid ounce), and sugars (partly inverted) 9·1 parts; the total solids amounted to 12·8 parts, thus leaving 2·0 parts of vegetable extract per 100 fluid parts. The concentrated compound solution of sarsaparilla in the *British Pharmacopœia* contains about 21 parts of solids in 100 fluid parts, so that it may be concluded that the amounts of extracts of "Sarsaparilla, Dandelion, Mandrake, Dock, Pipsissewa, Juniper Berries, and other valuable vegetable remedies" in this mixture were not large. The liquid had a somewhat aromatic odour and taste, in which oil of juniper could not be detected, nor was it recognizable on distillation; none of the other ingredients mentioned is capable of being identified in such a mixture. No alkaloid was present, and careful search for other likely ingredients gave only negative results. The mixture contained 19·6 per cent. by volume of alcohol.

HUGHES'S BLOOD PILLS.

These pills, made in Wales, are sold in boxes, price 1s. 1½d., containing 30 pills.

They were described on the label as "For all Blood, Skin, and Nerve Diseases." In a circular enclosed with the box there was a dissertation on the functions and composition of the blood, from which the following extracts, with all their capital letters, are taken

> The Blood being therefore the Life of the living Body, it stands to reason that if it is poisoned, you poison the whole system, and eventually destroy the life of the man. When the blood is chilled, or distempered through breathing impure air, unhealthy food, etc., it at once gets disturbed, and breeds disease in some form or other. This is the cause of Blast, Scurvy, Piles, Boils, King's Evil, Swollen Glands, Inflammation of the Eyes and Lids, Pains in the Sides, Back, and Kidneys, Cough, Bronchitis, Pleurisy, Rheumatism, Wounds in the Legs and Different Parts of the Body, all Scorbutic Affections, Cancer, Pimples on the Face, Neck, etc., and all Skin Eruptions, Chilliness, Headache, Indigestion, Fullness after Meals, Dyspepsia, Vomiting, Loss of Appetite, Consumption, Toothache, Neuralgia, Fits, St. Vitus's Dance, all Liver Complaints, Costiveness, Yellow Jaundice, Depression of Spirits, Stitches in the Sides, Fevers, Epidemics, Plagues, Gout, Nerve Diseases, Lumbago, Erysipelas, all kinds of Inflammation, and most Chest Diseases.
>
> The noted Pills, "Hughes's Blood Pills," act directly upon the Blood and Juices of all parts of the system, which they Strengthen and Purify. By so doing the Liver, Kidneys, Heart, Lungs, Stomach, Bowels, Brain and Nerves are renewed and toned to such a degree that their functions are perfectly performed, securing to the man healthy days.

Very lengthy directions were given for taking the pills for a variety of complaints, from which it appeared that the usual dose was one or two pills at night, or one three times a day.

The pills had a thin loose coating of French chalk; after removing this the average weight was 2 grains. Analysis showed the presence of no inorganic salts, except the usual small quantities of phosphate, sulphate, etc., found in the ash of most vegetable drugs. The pill contained a trace of oil of cloves and consisted of powdered drugs to the extent of about half its weight; ginger and cinchona were identified in this portion; a trace of alkaloid was extracted, showing the properties of the alkaloids of cinchona. A portion of the tissue, which appeared to be derived chiefly from a seed, could not be recognized, and a lengthy series of comparisons failed to identify it. The remainder of the pill was separated into two substances, which appeared to be aloes and jalap resin, but in each a mixture as this pill presented, the identity of these substances cannot be established with complete certainty. The proportions of the ingredients, also, can only be ascertained approximately; the following formula was indicated:

Aloes	0·7 grain.
Jalap resin	0·2 ,,
Powdered cinchona bark	0·3 ,,
,, ginger	0·2 ,,
Oil of cloves	Trace.

In one pill.

CHAPTER VI.

"REMEDIES FOR' GOUT, RHEUMATISM, AND' NEURALGIA.

THE medicines here described vary considerably in their nature, and to some extent in the complaints for which they are recommended, but no definite line can be drawn between them. Some are primarily for gout, but are recommended also for rheumatism; others are mainly for rheumatism, but are also recommended for gout and neuralgia; while others, again, are chiefly advertised for neuralgia and headache.

BLAIR'S GOUT AND RHEUMATIC PILLS.

These pills, which are a British product, are sold in boxes, price 1s. 1½d., and containing 14 pills.

They were described in a circular accompanying the box as:

The great and universal remedy for the immediate relief and cure of Acute and Chronic Gout, Rheumatism, Suppressed Gout, Rheumatic Gout, Gouty Skin Diseases, Bronchitis and Asthma, Sciatica, Lumbago, and Neuralgia, and as a preventive or prophylactic where the disease has a tendency to recur, or attacking any vital part, as the Stomach, Brain, or Heart.

Other extracts from this circular are:

In all cases of Gout, no matter of what length of standing, they not only give relief from the almost intolerable pain, but where the patient has kept his bed for months, *One Box will frequently carry off the attack* in two or three days—in many cases of extreme torture relief has been obtained in two or three hours . . . in those gouty skin affections, Psoriasis and Eczema, these Pills have no equal.

Blair's Gout and Rheumatic Pills are not only efficacious in curing Gout, but in all those diseases allied to it.

They never fail. They always cure.

Directions and Doses.

For Gout and Rheumatic Gout.—Take two Pills three times a day, just after meals, and when it is very severe, take two during the night, and they should be persisted in until the swelling and stiffness have disappeared.

In cases of long standing, where the tendency of the disease is to recur, it is advisable to take a short course of the Pills as a preventive. Dose.—Two twice a day for a fortnight.

For Suppressed Gout, including Gouty Asthma, Bronchitis, Dyspepsia Rheumatism, Rheumatic Headaches, Lumbago, Sciatica, Tic Doloreux, Pain in the Head, Face, etc., they must also be taken, two Pills three times a day, just after meals, that quantity being generally sufficient, but in some cases a longer continuance of them is necessary, particularly in Rheumatism of long standing, but that will also be eradicated by perseverance in the use of these Pills. *They should be taken from time to time also as a preventive.*

Spring and Autumn. In these treacherous Gout and Rheumatic Seasons, to prevent a recurrence, sufferers are earnestly advised to take a short alterative course of this famous medicine.

It is requested, in case this medicine should considerably open the bowels, that it may be laid aside until that effect has ceased, when it may be resumed, beginning with a smaller dose. Patients are also informed that it is unnecessary for any aperient medicine to be taken during its use, unless they have been costive for some days.

The pills had an average weight of 2·9 grains. Analysis showed them to contain powdered colchicum corm, exsiccated alum, and an excipient. The quantities found indicated the following formula:

Powdered colchicum corm	2.1 grains.
Burnt alum	0·35 grain.

in one pill.

The estimated cost of the ingredients for 14 pills is one-seventh of a penny.

HAMM'S RHEUMATIC, GOUT, AND SCIATICA CURE.

The Originator and Proprietor of this cure, who hails from the north of England, charges 2s. 9d. for a bottle containing 8 fluid ounces. It was described on the outside package as "The Greatest Remedy in the World. It has no equal for the cure of Rheumatism, Gout, and Sciatica." In a circular enclosed with the bottle it was stated that:

It never fails to Cure those distressing and torturing Complaints, and in most cases has given relief from the excruciating pains by taking a few doses. This Standard Remedy has time and again succeeded after all other internal remedies have failed. Purify the Blood by driving the Uric Acid from the system and you will remove the cause of all Rheumatism, etc. Hamm's Famous Rheumatism Cure has Never Failed to do it.

The dose was given on the label as "One Tablespoonful three times a day, after meals."

The preparation was a brown, slightly turbid liquid. Analysis showed it to contain potassium iodide, sodium salicylate, a little vegetable extractive, and a trace of alcohol. The extractive was moderately bitter, but possessed no characters indicating the drug from which it was derived; it contained no alkaloid. Quantitative determination of the ingredients showed the formula to be:

Potassium iodide	15 grains.
Sodium salicylate	66 ,,
Extractive	28 ,,
Alcohol	Trace.
Water to	8 fluid ounces.

Assuming the extractive to be of the same price as extract of gentian, the estimated cost of the ingredients of 8 fluid ounces is ½d.

GLORIA TREATMENT FOR RHEUMATISM.

This "treatment" is advertised as follows:

Cure yourself of Rheumatism. I will tell you how and send you the remedy Free. My combination treatment cures, not merely relieves but actually cures, cases of Rheumatism, Gout, and Sciatica. . . . The numerous so-called remedies offered to the public, through the medium of the newspapers, have absolutely killed all confidence; therefore, in order to make my genuine remedy more generally known, I have decided to give away a large quantity so that everybody can test for themselves the truth of my statements. My combination treatment consists of: 1. Gloria Balm, which Instantly Relieves Pain. 2. Gloria Pills which Purify the Blood and Invigorate the Whole System. 3. Gloria Tonic Tablets which Effect a Complete and Permanent Cure. . . . I earnestly ask every Rheumatic Sufferer to obtain a free supply of this medicine at once. Simply send a postcard request, and a supply will reach you in less than 24 hours.

Application to the address given brought sample boxes of the pills and tablets only, accompanied by a booklet entitled "Rheumatism and Gout, Causes and Cure," and a letter of the usual type, as indicated by the following extracts:

I was very pleased to receive your communication this morning, as having suffered from the terrible disease with which you are afflicted myself it naturally affords me a great deal of gratification to be able to place in the hands of every sufferer a genuine remedy for it—a remedy which cured me and has cured many thousands of others besides. . . .

It is, as I have often heard it described by persons bubbling over with gratitude for their relief from the above distressing ailments, Nature's very own cure for Rheumatism and Gout. The danger of allowing the poisonous acids which cause these diseases to continue their work day by day in the body cannot be exaggerated. . . .

Before closing this letter I once more beg to impress upon you the danger of delay in commencing the treatment, especially as applied to your particular case.

Since "Gloria Balsam" was apparently not thought sufficiently important for a sample to be sent, supplies were obtained of the tablets and pills only for examination.

Gloria Tonic, price 4s. 6d. a box, containing 50 tablets, was described on the box as "a scientific preparation for the cure of all uric acid ailments, including Rheumatism and Gout, Lumbago, Sciatica, Scrofula, and all other diseases resulting from Impurities of the Blood." This rather wide claim was somewhat at variance with statements made in the booklet, from which a few extracts may be given :

It was with the object of curing all rheumatism that I introduced "Gloria Tonic" to the public, and I believe that it is a task worthy of the cause. I do not propose to make the attempt with a remedy similar to the many thousands of cure-alls with which the market is overloaded, but with a true and reliable rheumatism specific—"Gloria Tonic."

I am not offering you a remedy of that kind, but one which is solely compounded for the cure of rheumatism, one that has been tested in Hospitals and Sanatoriums, one that has the endorsement of physicians and University professors, and, above all, one which has already enabled many hundreds of persons to abandon crutch and cane. Do not wonder if this can be true. The foregoing statement is an absolute fact. . . .

I could easily get many times 4s. 6d. for a box of "Gloria Tonic," but it is my purpose not so much to accumulate wealth as to benefit suffering mankind . .

"Gloria Tonic" is to-day the only remedy on the market that cures all forms of rheumatism effectively, and without destroying the delicate tissues of the Heart, Stomach, Liver, and Kidneys. . . .

The merit of this remedy is unapproachable. I have no object in telling you this aside from having your interests at heart, and wish to protect you against the many harmful drugs. You need not have any fear in taking "Gloria Tonic" as directed, while the smallest dose of other rheumatic remedies might harm you.

The directions were .

For adults: From one-half to one tablet is a dose, and four doses should be taken daily as follows: Half to one tablet before the morning, noon, and evening meal, and on retiring. . . . Dose for children from 10 to 15 years, one half-tablet. From 5 to 10 years, one-quarter of a tablet. Below these years, the medicine should not be given.

The average weight of the tablets was 11·2 grains; among 12 weighed separately the weights varied from 10·5 to 12·5 grains. Analysis showed the presence of potassium iodide, guaiacum resin, extract of liquorice, powdered liquorice, starch, mineral matter—apparently a mixture of talc and kaolin—a resinoid substance, and a trace of alkaloid. The alkaloid amounted to 0·016 per cent.; it did not agree in properties with any of the common alkaloids, but agreed, so far as it was practicable to examine it, with the alkaloid of phytolacca (the American weed, poke-root, or pokeberry); the resinoid also agreed in its properties with the resinoid phytolaccin, but there are no distinctive tests by which its identity could be certainly established. The quantities of the various ingredients were estimated as accurately as possible, and the following formula was indicated:

Potassium iodide	1·8 grains.
Guaiacum resin	0·8 grain.
Extract of liquorice	1·0 ,,
Resinoid (phytolaccin ?)....	0·9 ,,
Powdered liquorice	1·7 grains.
Rice starch	2·0 ,,
Talc and kaolin	2·1 ,,

In one tablet.

In the formula the most expensive ingredient is the phytolaccin, which is also the least certain, both as to identity and quantity. Taking the formula here given, the estimated cost of the ingredients for 50 tablets is 8d.

Gloria Pills, price 1s. 1½d. per box, containing 40 pills, in addition to being supplied as part of the "treatment" for rheumatism, were recommended as a general laxative. It was stated in the circular enclosed with them that "Gloria Laxative Pills will cure Constipation, Torpid Liver, Piles, Headache, Dizziness, Sour Eructation, Heartburn, Bloating, Flatulence, Nausea, Sleeplessness, Mental Depression, Palpitation of the Heart, Nervousness, Kidney Trouble, and all other conditions resulting from Dyspepsia and Indigestion."

The pills were coated with talc, coloured to a chocolate colour with oxide of iron. After removal of the coating, the average weight was 1·1 grains. Analysis showed the constituents to be chiefly extracts and resins. The two samples of pills examined—namely, the gratis sample of eight pills first supplied, and the full box afterwards obtained—differed materially in composition; the former contained about 25 per cent. of powdered liquorice, 6 or 8 per cent. of powdered rhubarb, and 6 or 8 per cent. of wheat flour, while the latter contained neither liquorice nor rhubarb, and proportionately more of the soluble constituents, which appeared to consist in both cases of extracts of aloes and cascara sagrada with jalap resin. The various constituents were estimated quantitatively, but in such a mixture exact results are of course unattainable, and even the qualitative results must be given with a certain reservation. The formula indicated for the pills in the 1s. 1½d. box was:

Extract of cascara sagrada	....	0·3 grain.
,, Socotrine aloes	....	0·5 ,,
Jalap resin	....	0·07 ,,
Flour } Excipient }	....	q.s.

in one pill.
Estimated cost of ingredients for 40 pills, ½d.

BARING GOULD'S ANTI-RHEUMATIC PEARLS.

This article is introduced to the public by an advertisement headed:

"Rheumatism speedily cured." The advertisement states that Mr. Baring Gould, of an address at a provincial watering place, "very strongly recommends Marvellous Cheap Remedy for Chronic Rheumatism, Gout, etc. Free Information for addressed envelope."

Application for information with regard to the remedy brought a box of the "Pearls" with an intimation that the price was 5s., or 3s. 9d. for prompt cash. In the enclosed circulars the proprietor was described as "W. Baring Gould, Rheumatic Specialist and Scientist in Chemistry," and the "Pearls" were referred to in the following terms:

Baring Gould's Anti-Rheumatic "Pearls" (Patent and Trade Mark Regis. tered). The Most Wonderful and Most Effectual "Anti-Rheumatic" Ever Known. . . .

Mr. Baring Gould desires to say that from a recent careful examination of his records, he finds that he relieves or cures (mostly by his wonderful "Pearls") at least eighty people in every hundred who come under his care.

There is nothing to approach the "Pearls" in Curative value for all kinds of Rheumatism, Sciatica, and Gout. They are entirely free from every kind of injurious substance, and may be taken with absolute safety and benefit by the most delicate bedridden sufferers.

DOSE.—Take 2 Pearls twice a day. Being flexible and tasteless they are easily swallowed, or the gelatine casing may be removed and the contents placed in half a wine-glass of water (hot or cold) and taken in that way. The flavour of the medicaments is agreeable to the palate and to the stomach also.

The "Pearls" consisted of gelatine capsules, of the flattened form known commercially as "perles," containing a white powder. The average weight of the contents was 5·9 grains, the contents of single capsules varying from 5·0 to 6·5 grains. It should be said that aspirin, a drug in very common use for rheumatism, is acetyl-salicylic acid. Analysis showed the powder to consist of:

Acetyl-salicylic acid....	85 per cent
Sugar of milk	15 ,,

The estimated cost of ingredients for 40 capsules is 1½d.

GOWER'S GREEN PILLS.

These pills, which cost 1s. 1½d. per box, containing 44 pills, were described in the advertisement as:

A real remedy for rheumatism, backache, muscular rheumatism, sciatica, gout, lumbago, cramps, stiffness of joints, kidney disorders, dropsical swellings, etc. These Pills act directly on the organic and muscular parts of the body, and bring instant relief to tired, aching, and painful muscles and joints.

In the circular enclosed with the pills it was stated that:

The ingredients . . . are known only to the proprietors. They are not to be found either in the *British Pharmacopœia* or in any surgery in the land. It was not your doctor's fault that he did not cure you, it was his misfortune— he did not know how. He had not these remedies in his possession. We offer you the opportunity of using them and recovering your health.

Gower's Green Pills, though an eminently scientific pill, do not act like magic. The days of miracles have gone by. They act surely, but sometimes slowly in cases of Rheumatism of long standing.

In taking these pills we would like it to be thoroughly known that if your disease is one of long standing you cannot be completely cured with one or two boxes. A rheumatic sufferer who has tried most remedies and has been tortured with pain for five years cannot expect to be a new man in five weeks. If it takes as many as a dozen 2s. 9d. boxes to cure a case like this, the sufferer cannot but consider it the best investment that he ever made in his life.

The directions were:

One dose to be taken three times a day, before or after meals. Three Pills are one dose.

The pills were coated with talc, with a small quantity of a green colouring matter. After removal of the coating the pills had an average weight of 1·2 grains. Analysis showed them to contain soap (about 36 per cent.), an alkaline salicylate (about 37 per cent.), extractive, and vegetable tissue. No alkaloid was present; the extractive was dark in colour, without bitterness or other characteristic taste, and showed no properties by which its source could be identified; microscopic examination of the tissue showed the presence of two powders, one of which agreed well in its characters with powdered cimicifuga root, while the other bore much resemblance to jalap, but not enough to warrant the statement that it was jalap. The total amount of vegetable powder was about 20 per cent., of which about one-third appeared to be cimicifuga; 11 per cent. of silicious ash was also present.

DR. COLLIE'S OINTMENT.

This ointment, supplied by a Scottish Company at the price of 1s. 9d. for a box containing 1¾ ounces, is advertised in the following terms:

Try Dr. Collie for Rheumatism. His ointment positively cures while you sleep. You don't rub it in, but apply just like a poultice. It draws out the cause of your trouble, and a speedy cure ensues. Try Dr. Collie's Ointment—Instant relief for Sciatica, Lumbago, and swollen joints.

It appeared, however, from a booklet sent with the ointment that rheumatism was only one among a large number of complaints for which the ointment was recommended; it was described on the label as:

A certain cure for Sprains, Bruises, Cuts, Burns, Chapped Hands, Eczema, Blood Poisoning, Whitlows, Sea Water Boils, Abscesses, Piles, Rheumatism, Sciatica, Lumbago, Pains in the Back and Loins, and all Sores and Ulcers of every description.

The directions for its use in rheumatism were:

First wash the part to be treated with warm water and soda, then thoroughly dry—(a quantity of the ointment may then be well rubbed in). Now get a piece of thick cotton cloth (old sheeting answers very well) or better still, chamois leather, spread the ointment thickly and apply like a poultice. When the dressing begins to get dry, take it off, and after scraping the cloth replace it with fresh ointment. The part may, after a dressing or two, begin to itch, and the skin, being stimulated, may come out in a humour. If so, do not be alarmed but persevere. This is a sure sign that the Ointment is doing its work, drawing out the deleterious matter, viz., Uric Acid Poison, from the body through the most natural of all channels, the pores of the skin. -

Analysis showed the presence of colophony resin, petroleum jelly, a little beeswax, and a fatty base. The colophony was accompanied by a small proportion of another substance of resinous nature, which appeared to be the altered resin to be found in the variety of colophony known commercially as "black resin"; a dark substance was also present which appeared to consist of the natural impurities of crude petroleum; the fatty basis showed generally the properties of a mixture of lard and tallow. A similar ointment was obtained by using the following formula :

Black resin	12 per cent.
Beeswax	2 ,,
Crude petroleum jelly	26 ,,
Tallow	20 ,,
Lard	40 ,,

Estimated cost of ingredients for 1¾ ounces, 1d.

ZOX.

Zox is a powder made by a Company with an address in London and the price charged is 1s. for a box containing eight powders. It was described on the wrapper as :

The most marvellous pain reliever. Instantly cures Toothache, Neuralgia, Head-ache, Sciatica, and all Nerve Pains. Pure, Harmless, not Aperient.

In a circular enclosed with the box directions were given for taking the powders for neuralgia, toothache, headache, sciatica, rheumatic and gouty pains, and influenza. For neuralgia the directions were :

One Powder should be taken when in pain, and should the enemy return, continue the Powders every four hours, for a few days. If very weak from continual pain, take a few doses of Zox Tonic ; this will give you speedy relief.

For rheumatic and gout pains :

Take one Zox Powder two or three times a day while pain is acute ; avoid beer and spirits of all kinds.

The average weight of the powders was 4½ grains, single powders in a box varying in weight from 4 to 6 grains. Analysis showed the powder to consist of acetanilide only.*

The estimated cost of the drug for eight powders is one-tenth of a penny.

OQUIT.

The vendors, a Company with a London address, sell tubes of 20 tablets for 1s. 1½d.

This is advertised as follows:

Neuralgia. Within 10 minutes of taking "Oquit" that frightful nerve-racking pain will be cured. One dose will convince you. Try it.

A pamphlet was enclosed with the package, headed "Oquit for Headaches and Nerve Pains, Headache, Neuralgia, Gout, Sciatica, Rheumatism, Lumbago, Influenza, Feverish Colds, Sea Sickness." A few extracts are here given:

Oquit . . . is made in strict accordance with a medical prescription from drugs which are daily prescribed by the most eminent physicians for the relief of nerve pains. There is nothing experimental about "Oquit." The drugs of which "Oquit" is composed are perfectly well known, and their claim to be regarded as unrivalled for the purpose has been rigidly tested and endorsed by the leading exponents of modern medicine. What is really unique about "Oquit" is the scientific proportion in which the constituent drugs are combined. It is a remarkable fact, and one which is attested by every medical man, that the action of a drug may be made effective or ineffective according to the manner in which it is prescribed. There are certain subordinate drugs which prepare the way, as it were, for the action of a principal drug, and the proportion between the ingredients of a prescription is of vital importance in relation to the effect produced. It is to this scientifically adjusted proportion that the remarkably beneficial results of "Oquit" are due. . . .

In the cure of Neuralgia, "Oquit" has proved eminently successful when taken in the same way as recommended for headache, with the addition that a third and further doses should be repeated, if found necessary, at intervals of three hours. . . .

In Rheumatism, whether the acute or chronic forms, "Oquit" is extremely beneficial, expelling from the system the inflammatory agents which give rise to the frequently excruciating pains in the joints and muscles involved, and confers a most welcome relief. . . .

In Gout, Sciatica, and Lumbago the eliminating power of "Oquit" is of the greatest possible value. In all these cases, adults should take three "Oquits" every three hours at the commencement of an attack, reducing the dose to two, and then to one, as the pain decreases.

The average weight of the tablet was 5·1 grains. Analysis showed them to contain:

Acetyl-salicylic acid	66·2 per cent
Starch, chiefly maize	20·0 ,,
Talc	4·2 ,,
Gum	1·5 ,,
Extractive	3·1 ,,
Moisture	5·0 ,,
Alkaloid	a trace.

As stated above aspirin is acetyl-salicylic acid, and so it may be added is xaxa.

The alkaloid did not show well-marked characters by which it could be identified, but agreed fairly well in its reactions with the total alkaloid of gelsemium; the general nature of the extractive was consistent with its being a preparation of this drug.

The estimated cost of ingredients for 20 tablets is ¾d.

GENOFORM TABLETS.

A substance was described under the name Genoform in the *Pharmaceutische Post* in 1905, as being the methylene-glycol ester of salicylic acid; but as the present preparation is advertised to the public, and supplied under a patent medicine stamp, it must be regarded as a secret remedy. The proprietor, it is stated, resides in Leipzig but there is a London agency, and the remedy is sold in tubes price 1s. 1½d., containing 10 tablets.

An advertisement of this preparation was headed: " Gout, Rheumatism, Sciatica, and Neuralgia Cured. A Miracle in Rheumatism." Then followed a testimonial describing the " miracle." On the package of the tablets it was stated that:

Genoform cures gout, rheumatism, sciatica, neuralgia, etc. Genoform gives instant relief and effects a permanent cure.

A circular enclosed in the package stated:

Genoform is a certain cure, and you need not suffer another day. No matter where the pain is, or how severe it is, or how long you have had it, Genoform Tablets will rid you of it. They give relief in many cases immediately, and produce a permanent cure.

Take them to-day and feel well. Genoform eases pain with a rapidity which is remarkable, at the same time doing away with the cause. Remember that.

It is no mere relief. It stamps out the cause of Gout, Rheumatism, Sciatica, and Neuralgia. It is absolutely harmless. No remedy equals it in its quick and certain effects.

Patients afflicted for years and unable to walk or use their limbs have been made sound and free from pain in a very little time. . . .

Absolutely crippled rheumatic persons, unable to dress or undress themselves, have entirely recovered with only a few doses of this preparation.

The directions were as follows:

The Tablets must never be taken on an empty stomach, but either during or after meals (from 3 to 9 tablets daily). Taking the Tablet is facilitated by letting it soak first in a spoonful of water and drinking a little water afterwards. Any oppression of the stomach is soon relieved by 5 or 6 drops of dilute Hydrochloric acid taken in half a glassful of water.

As Genoform contains Salicylic Acid and that well known drug for Rheumatism sometimes causes a little buzzing in the ears, if such buzzing ever occurs it is well to discontinue Genoform for 24 hours and afterwards take only a small dose for a day or so. It must be clearly understood that there is no possible harm or danger in such buzzing and few persons are so affected, but we think it wise to advise you lest you should think Genoform does not agree with you and discontinue its use.

The tablets had an average weight of 7·7 grains. They contained no free salicylic acid, but on hydrolysis with alkali they yielded 91·0 per cent. of that substance. Starch was present to the extent of 4·1 per cent., so that the material other than starch yielded 94·9 per cent. of its weight of salicylic acid. Salicyl-methylene-glycol ester $CH_2(C_7H_5O_3)_2$ would yield 95·6 per cent.; investigation of the other products of hydrolysis showed that this ester was the substance present; no other ingredient was found. On examination the substance proved to be hydrolyzed at once by alkali in the cold, but not by cold dilute acid; hot water caused slight decomposition, and on boiling it in water it readily yielded salicylic acid. The formula of the tablets is thus:

Salicyl-methylene-glycol ester	95 per cent.
Starch (and moisture)	5 "

POST'S C. B. Q. TABLETS FOR RHEUMATISM.

Two specimens of the proprietary article sold under the name of C. B. Q. have been examined at an interval of nine years. The earlier analysis showed that the tablets contained potassium iodide, quinine and colchicine in small quantities, a salicylate and extract of liquorice, used no doubt to bind the powder together. The analysis made in 1908 showed that of the tablets then examined each contained about 1½ grains of potassium iodide, a small quantity of salicylate, a vegetable extract, and magnesia. The extract was hygroscopic and the magnesia was no doubt employed to bring the mixture into a form suitable for tablet making. The extract was slightly bitter and the tablets contained a small amount of alkaloid, which was not certainly identified.

GOUT VARALETTES.

Analysis of Bishop's Gout Varalettes showed the presence of lithium citrate and a small quantity of what appeared to be piperazine, together with the usual effervescing basis consisting of sodium bicarbonate and tartaric acid.

PISTOIA GOUT POWDERS.

There was a powder for gout known to an earlier generation under the name of the "Portland Gout Powder;" according to the prescription given by Jourdan in the *Pharmacopée Universelle* (1828); it consisted of: Gentian root, round birthwort root (*Aristolochia rotunda*), ground pine root (*Teucrium chamaepitys*), the tops of germander (*Teucrium chamaedrys*), and of the lesser centaury (*Erithroea centaurium*), of each equal parts to be ground separately to a fine powder and mixed; dose, half a teaspoonful. He gives of this three variants, in one of which the gentian is replaced by guaiacum.

For some years past a good deal has been heard about the Pistoia gout powders. A pamphlet entitled *The antigouty powders of the R.R. Benedictine Mothers of Pistoia for the treatment of a gouty source* (Rome, 1904) presents a curious resemblance to the advertising pamphlets issued by ordinary nostrum dealers. There is a short disquisition on gout written in very odd English, this is followed by a translation of a large number of testimonials to the virtues of the powder, and this again by the following "Warning to our Customers":

> Having known that in some towns of Italy, and even in Pistoia, some antigouty drug circulates under the name of "Vegetal Antigouty Powders of the Cloister" or under other names alike, making every body trust that they come from our Monastery, we think ourselves, in duty bound, to remember to our Customers that no deposit of our Antigouty Powders is to be found neither in Pistoia nor in other towns or places in Italy or abroad, and that we have accorded to nobody the faculty of preparing or selling them.
>
> Consequently every antigouty remedy which in any way should be made known as coming from this Monastery, must be considered as a product of vulgar falsification and adulteration.

The label on some boxes of the powder states that it is based on gentian, and on Indian wood, which is one of the synonyms of guaiacum. The pamphlet, which has already been quoted, states that the powders do not contain colchicum, belladonna, or any other poisonous substance, but

are a composition of medicinal grasses, none of which can ever have a pernicious effect upon the health, whatever may be the state of the person who uses it,

It is asserted that "often many miraculous cures are obtained," but it appears that the treatment must be a prolonged one, for the pamphlet further states that:

When it is question of a first affection or of a light gouty attack, the treatment of a whole year without interruption can in general be sufficient; because it is necessary for the blood to stay under the action essentially depurative of the drug during four seasons.

But when the illness is old, a year of treatment cannot of course be enough to extirpate entirely the distemper, and the use of the drug must be protracted till necessary.

The sample of Pistoia gout powder examined was of a greenish ginger colour and had a bitter taste. MM. Guignard, Collin, Chastaing, and Barillot give the following formula for the Pistoia gout powder:

Colchicum corm	10 parts.
Bryony root	10 ,,
Betony (root, stem, and leaves)	50 ,,
Gentian root	10 ,,
Camomile (chiefly stem, leaves, a little root, and flowers)	10 ,,

M. Collin is one of the leading authorities on the microscopic characters of powdered vegetable drugs, and a microscopical examination of the specimen revealed characters consistent with this formula; such small differences as were observed were only such as might be expected between specimens grown under different conditions of soil, climate, etc.

Another formula which has been published for the powders is as follows, but the sample examined agreed more nearly with No. 1:

II.

Colchicum corm	20 parts.
Bryony root	10 ,,
Betony root	40 ,,
Gentian root	10 ,,
Camomile	10 ,,

LAVILLE'S ANTIGOUT REMEDIES.

According to Zernik, the chief constituents of the Liqueur du Dr. Laville, an antigout remedy, very popular in France, in spite of its high price and secret composition, are colchicin (about 0·08 per cent.) and quinine in alcoholic solution. The pilules du Dr. Laville are sold as preventive remedies against gout. They were found to contain extract of winter cherry, Physalis alkekengi, one of the Solanaceae (? capsicum), guaiacum resin, powdered leaves and root of the marsh mallow, and sodium silicate. Each bottle contains 75 grams, about $2\frac{1}{2}$ fluid ounces, and costs 8s.

SOME GERMAN NOSTRUMS.

The following notes upon a few German remedies are quoted from Dr. Zernik's reports in the *Deutsche Medicinische Wochenschrift*.

URICEDIN.

This is a Berlin product vaunted as a remedy for the gouty diathesis, but its composition is very simple; it contains $2\frac{1}{2}$ per cent. sodium chlorate, and 66·5 per cent. dry sodium sulphate, the remainder being sodium citrate and sodium tartrate.

RHEUMACID.

The prospectus asserts that this material, the result of years of careful and earnest study, revolutionizes all medical knowledge, and cures rheumatism, colds, neuralgia, sciatica, gout, bladder, kidney, and skin affections, etc. The price demanded for 50 grams (about $1\frac{1}{2}$ ounces) is 17s. 6d., while a sample costs 1s. The sample is supposed to contain ten doses of 1 gram each, but was actually found to contain only half that quantity. There appeared to be three sorts of rheumacid, marked A, B, and C respectively, but the analysis revealed that the constituents were practically the same and included aspirin, salol, and at times salpyrin, with a little citric acid. This seems rather like making a revolution with rosewater.

ANTIGOUT SOAP.

Lazarus Gout and Rheumatic Soap is prepared in Dresden. It is a piece of medium-quality sodium soap, containing a very small quantity of an ethereal oil. The cake weighs 70 grams (about 2 oz.), and costs 1 mark.

PINE PREPARATIONS.

Electricum, described as "aethereal Tyrolese fir and pine wood oil," and recommended by the vendors as an external remedy for rheumatism, gout, pains in the limbs, paralysis, sciatica, lumbago, and backache, neuralgia, tumours, etc., seems to consist merely of pine oil.

Weigand's Rheumatic and Gout Spirit which it is stated relieves the pain within a few hours and cures after a short time, consists of 55 parts of turpentine oil, 55 parts of spirits of camphor, and 5 grams of Venice soap. A bottle containing 115 grams, less than 4 ounces, costs 2s. 6d.

RHEUMA TABAKOLIN.

This is a Berlin preparation; a box containing about 100 grams (about 3½ oz.) costs 5s., but the quantity for neglected and obstinate cases cost 15s. It is asserted to be a newly discovered remedy for rheumatism and gout obtained from tobacco. The directions are to extract the material with about 24 ounces of 50 per cent. alcohol, and to use this extract as a liquid application to the painful areas. Analysis showed that the substance consisted of waste and powdered tobacco perfumed with lemon oil. In Germany waste broken tobacco can be bought at about 5d. or 6d. a pound.

CHAPTER VII.

KIDNEY MEDICINES.

This group of nostrums consists of those which are put forward for the cure of kidney troubles, or conditions of ill-health commonly, but as a rule erroneously, attributed by the public to kidney disease. Several of these are in the form of pills, while others are liquids. The two principal drugs employed are oil of juniper and potassium nitrate (nitre or saltpetre), separately or together; in some cases aperients are added. Altogether extravagant claims are made for some of the articles, as is usual, of course, with proprietary medicines; this point is dealt with more fully in the descriptions of individual preparations.

In analysing complex mixtures, such as some of these nostrums are, it is, of course, not possible to attain the same precision as when dealing with medicines which consist chiefly of inorganic salts, as in the case of nostrums for epilepsy, dealt with in another chapter. A vegetable extract containing no definite active principle, such as, for instance, extract of taraxacum (dandelion), cannot be identified by any direct test; if such an extract is mixed with another, with a powdered drug, or an essential oil, its identification with perfect certainty may become almost impossible. The large variations, again, which may occur in the proportion of solid matter in a tincture or infusion, as well as the variations in the relative proportion of the different constituents of drugs, prevent the results of analysis being translated with certainty into the formula from which the mixture was compounded. These considerations apply to several of the articles described in this chapter. While the principal ingredient or ingredients in each case can be ascertained with little or no possibility of error, the subsidiary ingredients in some cases cannot be determined with the same confidence; we have endeavoured to indicate in each case the possibility of such minor errors. Full use has been made of check methods, by compounding mixtures according to the formulæ obtained by analysis and comparing them with the originals.

DOAN'S BACKACHE KIDNEY PILLS.

These pills, of American origin, which have been very extensively advertised for some years, are sold in boxes price 2s. 9d., containing 40 "kidney pills" and 4 "dinner pills."

They were described on the wrapper of the package as a

> Specific for kidney complaints and all diseases arising from disorder of the kidneys and bladder. Cure Backache, Weak Back, Rheumatism, Diabetes, Congestion of the Kidneys, Inflammation of the bladder, Gravel, Bright's Disease, Scalding Urine, and all Urinary troubles.

A circular was enclosed with the box, in which a dissertation on "Diseases of the Kidneys and Bladder" was given, together with directions for taking the pills for various complaints. The following extracts are taken from the circular:

> Doan's Backache Kidney Pills are composed of rare and valuable medicina agents in a combination best adapted to the speedy relief and cure of Kidney Disease, urinary and bladder affections, and all diseases resulting therefrom. They are purely vegetable, containing no ingredients of a deleterious nature, and may be taken by the most delicate person, with every confidence of their giving quick and permanent relief, without any after ill effects. . . . they are the only medicine known that quickly relieves and permanently cures.
>
> This medicine has restored to health thousands of women. As a means of healing the kidneys, and as a tonic to the whole female constitution it is unequalled.

The last sentence of the next extract shows some ingenuity:

> Chronic cases of long standing. These frequently come under our notice and we hear that the patient, after trying every known remedy and failed (sic) has despaired of ever getting relief. Now in all stages of Kidney Disease this is where Doan's Backache Kidney Pills are the most needed, and, indeed, are the only remedy possible to give permanent relief. But it takes time. One cannot expect to be cured in a few weeks. . . In some cases three or four boxes of Doan's Backache Kidney Pills are sufficient; but in these cases of long standing, 8, 10, and even 20 or 30, are required to effect a cure. But they will cure in the end if the patient perseveres. We are emphatic on this point, because in kidney disease patients are so easily discouraged. It is one of the symptoms of the disease.

The directions were to take from two to four of the dinner pills at night before commencing to take the kidney pills; then to begin with one kidney pill after each meal and one at bedtime, increasing the dose to two or three, after a short time. For children under 8, the dose was given as half a pill after each meal and at bedtime.

The "kidney pills" were ovoid in shape, and of a brown-grey colour externally, with sugar-coating beneath the thin, coloured layer; after removing the coating, the average weight of the pills was about 2 grains. Analysis showed them to contain oil of juniper and (in spite of their "purely vegetable" nature) potassium nitrate, together with a considerable proportion of a resinous substance, and of powdered fenugreek seeds and wheat and maize starches. Examination of the resin showed it to be derived from a coniferous source, and on comparison with various coniferous resins it agreed in characters with that of *Abies canadensis* (*Pinus canadensis*), known as hemlock pitch. The proportions of the different ingredients were determined by analysis; but oil of juniper, in such small quantity, can only be approximately determined, and the amount found was confirmed by comparison of a pill containing this quantity with the pill under examination. The following formula gives a similar pill:

Oil of juniper	1 drop.
Hemlock pitch	10 grains.
Potassium nitrate	5 ,,
Powdered fenugreek	17 ,,
Wheat flour	4 ,,
Maize starch	2 ,,

In twenty pills.

The estimated cost of the materials of the 40 kidney pills and 4 dinner pills, ½d.

The dinner pills, of which four were included in the box of kidney pills, are also supplied separately in boxes of 50 for 1s. 1½d. The label stated that:

Doan's Dinner Pills Cure Constipation, Sick Headache, Biliousness, Dizziness, and all deranged conditions of Stomach, Liver, and Bowels.

The directions were:

For adults, 1 to 3 Pills; for children, ¼ to 1 Pill.

These statements and directions were amplified in a handbill enclosed in the package.

The pills were ovoid and enclosed in white sugar coating; the average weight of one, without coating, was about ¾ gr. Analysis showed the presence of podophyllin, aloin, oil of peppermint, a resin that appeared to be jalap resin, cayenne, liquorice, gum, maize starch, and a small quantity of an extract that resembled extract of henbane; as the extract last named had no sufficiently well-marked characters to enable a small quantity of it to be distinguished perfectly when mixed with larger quantities of the other drugs named, the identity of this ingredient could not be completely established. The following formula gives a similar pill:

Oil of peppermint	1 drop.
Podophyllin	3·8 grains.
Aloin	6·9 ,,
Jalap resin	0·8 grain.
Powdered capsicum	0·5 ,,
,, liquorice	0·6 ,,
Maize starch	0·5 ,,
Acacia gum	1·5 grains.
Extract of henbane	1·5 ,,

(In twenty pills.)

Estimated cost of materials of 50 pills, 1d.

DODD'S KIDNEY PILLS.

These pills, made by an American Company advertising from a London address, are sold in boxes containing 35, price 2s. 9d.

The label round the box stated:

A positive cure for all kidney diseases: cures rheumatism, Bright's disease, diabetes, back-ache; cures female weakness, purifies the blood, cleanses the system.

The following extracts are from a circular enclosed with the pills:

Experience has proved that Dodd's Kidney Pills are the only cure for kidney diseases.

Dodd's Kidney Pills is the only remedy that has cured Bright's Disease.

Diabetes—Dodd's Kidney Pills will cure this disease.

Dropsy—The first object in treating dropsy is to restore the kidneys to their normal condition. This is what Dodd's Kidney Pills do and hence their peculiar efficacy for this disease.

Dodd's Kidney Pills will cure any form of heart disease.

What is known as the "change of life," is a period of great importance to woman. At such a time, no remedy could be more effective than Dodd's Kidney Pills.

These pills . . . consist of the active principles of vegetable substances which have been carefully studied by the discoverer of the remedy, both as to their nature and effect, and finally given to the world in the form of a sugar-coated pill, which to-day is universally acknowledged to be the best kidney remedy obtainable.

The directions are:

Take one to three pills morning, noon, and night, before or after meals. In the majority of cases one pill is a dose.

The pills were ovoid in shape, coated and coloured red on the outside. The colouring matter formed a strongly fluorescent yellow solution, showing it to be fluorescein or an allied substance; the coating was of sugar on the outside, with an inner layer consisting of chalk. In spite of the statement quoted above, that the pills consist of the active principles of vegetable substances, it was no surprise to find that the principal ingredient was potassium nitrate, of which each contained about 1 gr.; the other constituents were sodium bi-carbonate, soap, hard paraffin, wheat flour, powdered turmeric, two resins respectively soluble and insoluble in ether, a small quantity of a bitter substance, and a little extractive. Examination of the resins showed that they agreed in their characters with the two constituents of jalap resin; the bitter substance was not alkaloidal, and after careful comparison with a large number of bitter principles was found to agree with that of cascarilla. The following formula gives a pill which is practically identical with the one under examination:

Extract of cascarilla (alcoholic)	0·15 grain
Jalap resin	0·3 ,,
Hard soap	1·0 ,,
Potassium nitrate	1·0 ,,
Sodium bicarbonate	0·85 ,,
Hard paraffin	0·5 ,,
Turmeric	0·3 ,,
Wheat flour	0·8 ,,
In one pill.	

The estimated cost of the materials of 35 pills is 1d.

Dr. VAR'S AMERICAN KIDNEY PILLS.

On the outside of the package these pills, which are advertised from an address in a town in the south of England, and sold in boxes of 14 costing 1s. 1½d., are stated to "correct the stomach and stimulate the liver and kidneys." In a circular enclosed with the box they are referred to as "Certain Corrective! Positive Cure!" while the obscurity of the following is perhaps intended to make the warning conveyed more effective:

Do not let slight or severe Kidney Disorders develop into Cancerous Decay, Twin Complaints—Kidney Liver Diseases. Cure them! Put both in strong active order. There is not a safer, surer, speedier remedy in existence. Myriads of people thank Providence for Dr. Var's Kidney Pills. *Should be taken for Natural Weak Kidneys.*

The directions are:

One to be taken three times a day after meals.

The "pills" were in reality flexible capsules, each containing about 5½ grains of a soft mass in which oils of juniper and peppermint could be recognized in small quantity; examination also showed the presence of potassium nitrate, of small quantities of iron and magnesium compounds, and of lycopodium,* together with powdered squill, wheat starch, and a "green" extract, containing a trace of alkaloid, which appeared from its characters to be a mixture of extracts of henbane and taraxacum. The iron was perhaps an accidental impurity, and the magnesia and lycopodium were probably added to assist in making up the mass and **not** for therapeutic effect. The following formula gives a similar mass:

Oil of peppermint	1 drop.
„ juniper	8 drops.
Potassium nitrate	8 grains
Powdered squill	3 „
Wheat flour	6 „
Extract of henbane	7 „
„ taraxacum	21 „

In 10 capsules.

The estimated cost of the materials of 14 capsules is under ⅜d.

FITCH'S KIDNEY AND LIVER COOLER.

A bottle of this preparation containing rather less than 4 fluid ounces is sold for 2s. The directions are:

Take two teaspoonfuls mixed in water every morning.

---

* Lycopodium is a fine powder consisting of plant-spores sometimes used by pharmacists for enveloping pills which easily take up moisture.

The label and package appear to have been devised for the purpose of suggesting, without explicitly stating, that it is a cure for the complaints named. On one side appears the following (divided into sections by use of different type):

Oh my back, how it aches! Why? Fitch's Kidney and Liver-Cooler. Trade Mark. Sluggish liver. Inactive kidneys. Over-heated blood. Bad urine. Acts chemically by absorption.

and on the other:

Oh my back, how it aches! Why? Because your Kidneys and Liver are Sluggish, and a deposit has formed in the urine which will contaminate the whole system unless dissolved chemically. Try this; you won't regret. It's a grand conception.

Analysis showed the liquid to consist simply of a solution of potassium nitrate in water, the strength being 56 grains in a fluid ounce—that is, 14 grains in a dose.

The estimated cost of the contents of the bottle is one-eighth of a penny.

WARNER'S "SAFE" CURE.

Warner's Safe Cure is a liquid sold in a bottle holding about 8 fluid ounces at the price of 2s. 9d.

The label bore the words, "For Kidney and Liver and Bright's disease and jaundice, gravel, stone"—and a long list of other complaints. "Dose for adults, one tablespoonful 5 or 6 times a day."

A "medical pamphlet" of 34 pages accompanied the bottle, from which the following extracts are taken:

Warner's "Safe" Cure is a purely vegetable compound, and contains no narcotic or harmful drugs; it is free from sediment and is pleasant to take; it is a most valuable and effective tonic; it stimulates digestion, awakens the torpid liver, and puts the entire system in the very best receptive state for the work of restoring the kidneys. It does its work with absolute method, preparing the tissues, soothing and stimulating the enfeebled organs, healing at the same time. It builds up the body, gives it strength, and restores the energy which is or has been wasting under the baneful suffering of kidney disease. Warner's "Safe" Cure was discovered about thirty years ago by one of the most eminent specialists in diseases of the kidneys, who had made a life-study of kidney and kindred diseases.

How to test your kidneys. Put some morning urine in a glass or bottle; let it stand for twenty-four hours; if there is a reddish sediment in the bottom of the glass, or if the urine is cloudy or milky, or if you see particles or germs floating about in it, your kidneys are diseased and you should lose no time but get a bottle of Warner's "Safe" Cure, as it is dangerous to neglect your kidneys for even one day. Bright's disease, gravel, liver complaint, pains in the back, rheumatism, rheumatic gout, inflammation of bladder, stone in the bladder, uric acid poison, dropsy, eczema, scrofula, blood disease, offensive odour from sweating, so-called ' female weakness,' painful periods, too frequent desire to urinate, and painful passing of urine are all caused by diseased kidneys, and can be speedily cured by Warner's " Safe " Cure, which has been prescribed for twenty-five years."

Of Bright's disease it is remarked:

It is one of the harassing complaints which physicians in family practice seldom have the patience to investigate and manage with sufficient care.

The assumed predilection of the public for vegetable remedies is no doubt answerable for potassium nitrate being classed as " purely vegetable " in so many of these medicines. In the present case analysis showed the presence of potassium nitrate, alcohol, glycerine, a trace of oil of wintergreen, and vegetable extractive; there was no alkaloid or similar active principle, and the extract had little distinctive taste or character; all its properties pointed to its consisting largely of extract of taraxacum, with some other extract containing a small quantity of tannin; a careful series of comparisons with all the drugs in ordinary use which were not excluded by various tests did not identify it with any of them, and it is probable that it is obtained from some non-medicinal plant.

The following formula gives an almost identical mixture:

Potassium nitrate	50 grains.
Oil of gaultheria	¼ minim.
Rectified spirit	5 fluid drams.
Liquid extract of taraxacum	10 ,,
Glycerine	4 ,,
Water to	8 fluid ounces.

This contains about 10 per cent. of pure alcohol, which is the proportion found in Warner's Cure; in a mixture of which a tablespoonful was to be taken five or six—or, according to the handbill with it, six to eight—times a day, this proportion of alcohol is by no means negligible.

In such a mixture there is no means of determining exactly the amount of liquid extract of taraxacum, especially as it is liable to vary considerably in colour and in amount of solid residue; this is by far the most expensive ingredient in the above formula, and it is probable that the amount is here over-estimated. Taking the quantity here given, the estimated cost of the drugs for one bottle of the mixture is 5¼d.

VENO'S SEAWEED TONIC.

The Company in Manchester which advertises Veno's Seaweed Tonic sells it at the price of 1s. 1½d. a bottle, holding 2¾ to 3 fluid ounces.

The label states:

Contains in a pleasant and agreeable form the active principles of seaweed. First introduced into the medical world by Mr. Veno, and now admitted to be a most efficient and valuable medicine. Veno's seaweed tonic is prepared on an entirely new principle, and is free from poisonous or mineral drugs. It cures all ailments arising from a diseased condition of the Stomach, Liver, Kidneys, and Blood, which, when diseased, cause nearly all sickness. Dose.—For an adult, one teaspoonful twice or three times daily.

The following extracts are taken from a pamphlet enclosed with the bottle:

Veno's Seaweed Tonic is a specific remedy; money cannot make it better. If it fails, no other medicine will ever succeed; but sufferers must have patience.

Kidney Diseases, Weak Back, Backache or Lumbago, Incipient Bright's Disease. If you suffer from a weak back, with pain, soreness, or stiffness; if there is a dragging weakness in the limbs and lack of muscular energy; or if your urine is very clear or high coloured, showing a sediment of white flakes through it, it indicates a weakness or disease of the kidneys. Veno's Seaweed Tonic should be taken for at least two or three months, in teaspoonful doses twice or three times daily, after meals.

The mixture contained a small proportion of undissolved sediment, which, when collected and examined, agreed in all respects with the insoluble portion of leptandrin. Glycerine, a little phosphate, alcohol, and a trace of chloroform were present, and vegetable extractive. Careful examination of the latter gave evidence of the presence of the constituents of cascara sagrada, senna, and rhubarb. Such a mixture as this could not, of course, be quantitatively resolved into its components, and the proportions given below were arrived at by comparisons of the properties of various trial mixtures with the properties of the original; no indication was obtained of any substance derived from seaweed. The following formula gives a practically identical mixture:

Leptandrin	10 grains.
Sodium phosphate, crystals	33 ,,
Liquid extract of cascara sagrada....	45 minims.
Concentrated infusion of rhubarb (1–7)	1 fluid dram.
,, ,, senna (1–7)	2½ fluid drams.
Glycerine	2 ,,
Chloroform water	1 fluid ounce.
Water to	3 fluid ounces.

The estimated cost of the ingredients is 1½d.

MUNYON'S KIDNEY CURE.

This is sold by Munyon's Homoeopathic Home Remedy Company from an address in London, but is stated to be "Manufactured in U.S. of America." The price is 1s. a bottle, containing 132 pilules.

The directions are: "Four pellets every hour," which must at least keep the patient amused.

The label bears the words:

Cures Bright's disease, gravel, all urinary troubles, and pain in the back or groins from kidney diseases.

The following extracts are from a circular enclosed with the bottle:

Munyon's Improved Homœopathic Remedies are radically different from those used by the regular school of homœopathy or any other system of medicine. We have the true cure for the most obstinate as well as the most intricate of diseases. The whole secret of Munyon's Remedies is the science of combining and harmonizing all drugs that are known to cure certain diseases, so that by our special combinations we cover every phase of the case, no matter what the complaint. There is no experimenting, no guesswork, but an absolutely fixed law of cure.

Munyon's Kidney-Cure has no equal. It cures pain in the back, loins, or groins, from kidney disease, puffy and flabby face, dropsy of the feet and limbs, frequent desire to pass water, scanty urine, dark-coloured and turbid urine, sediment in the urine, gravel in the bladder, and too-great a flow of urine.

The pilules were found to vary much in size, the average weight being 0·6 grain. Analysis showed them to consist of ordinary white sugar; no trace could be detected of any alkaloid or other active principle, or of any medication. The sugar was determined quantitatively, and found to be just 100·0 per cent. of the weight of the pilules.

Estimated cost of contents of bottle, one thirty-fifth of a penny.

CHAPTER VIII.

DIABETES.

DIABETES, being a disease which runs on the whole a steady course unaffected by anything but diet, does not afford a promising field for the use of drugs; but as drowning men catch at straws, patients who have been told that they are incurable are naturally disposed to try any remedy that holds out a prospect of cure or relief. Although there are a good many proprietary remedies for diabetes, few seem to have a large sale, but such as exist are pushed by the usual pretensions set forth in advertisements and circulars. Every one must admit that few things can be more cruel than to trade upon the hopes and fears of sick people or to sell them worthless remedies with the positive assurance of cure. Yet this is what is done by the sellers of quack remedies, and the Inland Revenue pockets the patent medicine duty without a blush. Some account is here given of two much advertised preparations—Vin Urané Pesqui and Dill's Diabetic Mixture. It may be objected that Pesqui's Uranium Wine is not a secret remedy because it is said to contain uranium nitrate, pepsin, and " other appropriate elements " added to " old Bordeaux wine " ; but uranium nitrate is a drug well known to the medical profession, and whatever may be its properties it is not a cure for diabetes. There is no trustworthy evidence that it has ever cured a single case, and the most that can be honestly said of it is that patients have improved in general health while taking it, although it has not influenced the amount of sugar. Yet we are told in this advertisement that Pesqui's Uranium Wine " positively cures sugared diabetes provided it is resorted to at an early stage and used during a sufficient length of time." Dill's Diabetic

Mixture appears to consist mainly of extract of hydrastis, a well-known drug, which amongst the many virtues claimed for it has never been shown to possess any influence over diabetes; yet the advertisement says that Dill's Diabetic Mixture is the "only known remedy for this deadly disease"! There is another triple nostrum for diabetes which, on examination, was found to consist of tablets of aspirin, unsweetened lime-juice, and a pink powder composed of sodium sulphate flavoured with oil of peppermint and tinted with phenol-phthalein. These simple remedies were solemnly vouched for by the vendors in the following words: "We have satisfied ourselves that the treatment is an absolute and permanent cure"! Apparently the law cannot reach those who publish deliberately untruthful statements with the object of selling their goods. The words of the judgment of the Lord Justice Clerk in a case with reference to Bile Beans, heard on appeal in the Court of Session at Edinburgh, should have aroused the Government to a sense of its duty to provide protection to the public. The Lord Justice Clerk exposed in plain language the procedure by which the vendors of this nostrum had worked up their business and palmed off their medicine on the public, yet the number of their advertisements does not appear to have diminished.

VIN URANÉ PESQUI.

This medicated wine is made in Bordeaux but is sold in this country from a depôt in London. The price charged for a bottle holding 24 fluid ounces is 8s.

A small booklet, entitled *Diabetes and its Cure by the Vin Urané Pesqui*, was enclosed with the bottle; a few extracts from this are here given:

It has been shown by medical statistics that there are in France every year 10,000 deaths or more, due to diabetes through a deficient treatment, whilst they could have been cured by taking the Vin Urané Pesqui. . . .

Organic sugar enters the blood together with the alimentary sugar, the former being destroyed by the molecular changes that it undergoes for the nutrition of the different organs. If not sufficiently destroyed, it is productive of glycohemia, and as it passes into the urine it brings forth glycosuria; this pathological state determines, in course of time, particularly among persons suffering from obesity, some of the following diseases: polydipsy (excessive thirst), oedema in the legs, the enfeeblement of the physical and intellectual faculties, visionary troubles, amblyopia, cataract or gutta-opaca, headaches and anaemia, followed by dryness of the skin, successive furuncles, gatherings or boils, eczemas, itching on the skin provoking an irresistible desire to scratch one self, anthrax, urinary gravel, lumbago, sciatica, albuminuria, polyuria (insipid diabetes, without sugar, excessive emission of urine), rheumatism, dropsy, bulimia (insatiable appetite) or polyphagia, azoturia (large quantity of urine with a heavy percentage of uric acid), then fearful complications; pneumonia, prurience, either vulvar or prepucial; diabetic phimosis, gangrene in different parts of the body, particularly in the toes, the nails of which become black; consumption, etc. Great mental worries are also productive of glycosuria. . . .

Pesqui's Urané Wine positively cures sugared diabetes, provided it is resorted to at an early stage and used during a sufficient length of time.

As soon as the patient has made use of this wine, his thirst is allayed almost instantaneously; his strength reappears; all his functions are gradually restored; his breathing, which the absence of feculents had rendered difficult, becomes easier; he is no longer put out of breath, nor does he feel any lassitude; he can now walk about without undergoing any fatigue; his look improves and his temper assumes a more pleasant character. . . .

The Vin Urané (Uranated Wine) prepared by Mr. Pesqui, of Bordeaux, has been qualitatively analysed at the Barral chemistry laboratory. The result of this analysis points to this medicine being a compound of old Bordeaux wine, in accordance with Bouchardat's prescriptions, to which the following elements have been added: azotate of uranium, pepsine, and other appropriate elements.

The dose was given on the label as .

Three small sherry-glassfuls per day, with or without water, 5 minutes before, or immediately after meals, and at night before bedtime.

Analysis of the wine showed it to contain, in 100 parts by measure:

Alcohol	8·75 parts.
Glycerine	3·55 ,,
Total solids	2·92 ,,
Fixed acid, reckoned as tartaric	0·43 part.
Volatile acid, reckoned as acetic	0·21 ,,
Reducing sugar	0·28 ,,
Cane sugar	doubtful trace.
Ash	0·30 part.
Uranium, equivalent to crystalline uranium nitrate	0·02

No digestive power whatever on egg-albumen could be detected, indicating the absence of unchanged pepsin. The amount of uranium found corresponds to one-twelfth of a grain of the nitrate in 1 fluid ounce, or half a grain in the daily dose, a sherry glass usually holding about 2 ounces.

The cost of the preparation depends, of course, on the cost of the original wine, and is scarcely affected by the added ingredients.

DILL'S DIABETIC MIXTURE.

This mixture is sold by a firm in Manchester at the price of 8s. 3d. for three bottles (not supplied singly), holding 2 fluid ounces each.

It was advertised in the following terms:

DIABETES.

Dill's Diabetic Mixture is the only known remedy for this deadly disease. No dieting necessary. It also cures Yellow Jaundice, Gall Stones, Hepatic Asthma, and all Liver Complaints. It is also the very best remedy we know for Kidney Diseases.

In a leaflet enclosed in the package it is stated:

In Diabetes the Government returns of health show that 100 per cent. die of the disease—that is, all of them—66 out of every 100 die of Coma, and 34 of Pneumonia, so that in ordinary medicine there is no cure. But after 15 years' experiment I discovered this remedy, by means of which hundreds have been restored to health and strength, the world and their families. It is the only known remedy for this deadly disease. . . .

. . . all Liver complaints and Kidney complaints are cured by this remedy. And it is natural that it should be so, for when we know that the Liver is the workshop of the body; that it makes the Blood, and the Bile, and the Urine, and the Sugar which the kidneys only filter out, I say, when we know this, we may be quite sure that any remedy that cures the liver benefits the whole body. The nerves, the flesh, the skin, the blood, and tissues; even the special senses such as sight, hearing, and smell, with the sense of touch are all improved and benefited by it.

The Remedy, it is needless to say, will have to be persevered with. These are deadly diseases and must have time.

The dose was given on the label as:

One teaspoonful every four hours in a tablespoonful of water.

The mixture contained a considerable amount of sediment, partly of a heavy nature and partly very light; this caused some difficulty in dividing the contents of a bottle without altering the relative proportions of the ingredients, and increased the possible error in the quantitative results. Alcohol was present to the extent of 35 per cent.; the heavier sediment consisted of sodium bicarbonate, which is very little soluble in such a liquid; this constituent formed 7·4 per cent. of the mixture. Two alkaloids were present in approximately equal proportions, the total amounting to 0·25 per cent.; these proved to be hydrastine and berberine, and the general nature of the extractive, etc., present showed that they had been added in the form of extract, fluid extract, or tincture of hydrastis; there is no official standard for the alkaloidal strength of these, but, taking the usual proportion, the alkaloid found would represent 1·5 per cent. of extract of hydrastis. This left a portion of the total solids to be accounted for; a small amount of a resin was found which resembled scammony resin in its properties, and a larger proportion of a resinoid having general resemblance to caulophyllin (obtained from the blue cohosh or squaw-root), but the identity of the resin and resinoid could not be established owing to the absence of characteristic properties. The formula was thus found to be:

Sodium bicarbonate	7·4 parts.
Extract of hydrastis	1·5 ,,
Resin, resinoid, and other extractive	2·2 ,,
Alcohol	35 ,,
Water to	100 ,,

On the rather liberal assumption that the whole of the unidentified portion costs as much as caulophyllin, the estimated cost of the ingredients for 6 fluid ounces is 11d.

A LANCASHIRE NOSTRUM.

A treatment for diabetes was, and perhaps is still advertised by a firm of manufacturing chemists in Manchester. In a letter addressed to an enquirer the manufacturers wrote:

The treatment was recently discovered by a Lancashire doctor who had himself suffered from diabetes for a great number of years, and used all the recognized medical treatments without effect. His own discovery cured him entirely. The formulas have been entrusted to us, and we are manufacturing and offering the preparation to the suffering public. We have satisfied ourselves that the treatment is an absolute and permanent cure. ׃ ׃ ׃ We have, therefore, every confidence in recommending it to you.

These statements are supported by a batch of testimonials which are not so strong as is usual in such cases. For example, one is headed in black type, "Completely cured a gentleman and his two friends," and runs as follows:

> Dear Sir,—I received the treatment yesterday. A friend of mine, a London gentleman, has told me your treatment and the Gluten Bread has (*sic*) completely cured him and two friends of his of sugar diabetes."

The medicines supplied consisted of (1) tablets, of which four were to be taken each morning, and (2) a mixture. A month's supply was forwarded for 10s. 6d., from two to four months' treatment being said to be sufficient. A booklet was also sent giving the usual directions for a diet free from carbohydrates, and enjoining the use of warm clothing, with occasional hot or Turkish baths. The tablets (1) contained 5 grains of aspirin; the mixture (2) was composed of unsweetened lime-juice containing 6 per cent. of free citric acid. A pink powder, described as an aperient, consisted of dried sodium sulphate, flavoured with oil of peppermint, and tinted with phenolphthalein. These remedies are not new, nor has their use been attended with any particular success in the treatment of diabetes. It is difficult to see why they should give better results when supplied as a nostrum than when ordered in the usual way by medical men, unless we attribute something to the suggestive power of bold assertions and public advertisement.

NOTE ON DIABETIC FOODS.

In the treatment of diabetes it is the rule, in order to diminish the amount of sugar passed, to decrease or altogether exclude starchy foods from the dietary, and to replace them by various substitutes, of which the most important are gluten bread and biscuits. Some of the so-called gluten flour and special foods sold as suitable for diabetic patients are impositions, inasmuch as they are found to contain either as much or nearly as much starch as ordinary flour. In one instance brought to notice at the end of 1905, a so-called gluten flour and special diabetic foods obtained from Messrs. H. H. Warner and Co., Ltd., who are also the vendors of Warner's Safe Cure, but who in this instance acted as agents, it was found that the flour was practically ordinary wheaten flour. This is indicated in the following table, in which the result of the analysis of the special articles is placed side by side with the figures of the official analysis of wheaten flour published by the United States Department of Agriculture:

	Department of Agriculture, U.S.A.		The Special Materials.	
	Spring Wheat.	Winter Wheat.	Gluten Flour.	Special Diabetic Food.
Water....	10·4	10·5	12·65	11·06
Proteid	12·5	11·8	10·60	12·40
Fat	2·2	2·1	—	3·00
Convertible carbohydrates	71·2	72·0	70·30	71·06
Mineral matter	1·9	1·8	0·44	1·52
Fibre	1·8	1·8	—	—

It will be seen that the amount of starch and other convertible carbohydrates in spring wheat is 71·2, and in the so-called gluten flour 70·30.

CHAPTER IX.

OBESITY CURES.

THE claims made for nostrums advertised for the reduction of corpulence are, as a rule, rather less extravagant than usual. A reason for this is not far to seek; it is important that the consumer of the medicine shall be encouraged to persist in its use for a considerable time, and statements as to rapid cure might very soon be found to be at variance with the facts and would probably only lead to discontinuance of the medicine, and therefore defeat the maker's object. Nevertheless, the emphatic and confident statements, backed by testimonials, so important a weapon of the nostrum vendor, are by no means abandoned, as some of the quotations below will show. The prices named for the various articles described refer, as a rule, to the smallest size of package; in most cases larger packages, containing sufficient for several weeks' or months' consumption, are supplied at proportionally lower rates, and purchasers are urged to obtain these larger packages.

While certain of these preparations present no particular difficulty to the analyst, the majority not only contain vegetable preparations devoid of well-marked characters, but since the most important of these, extract and fluid extract of *Fucus vesiculosus*, are not prepared according to any official formula, and are naturally therefore liable so great variation, it is not possible to arrive with perfect certainty at the precise composition of such articles by analysis; and when, as in the case of any nostrum, the maker can draw on all unofficial and even non-medicinal substances for his ingredients, it is inevitable that some shall remain not certainly identified. It may fairly be assumed, however, that such unknown substances, possessing no well-defined chemical characters, will not be likely to have much, if any, therapeutic importance.

The belief that sucking lemons will make one thin is widespread, and gave origin a few years ago to a passing fashion, so that it was impossible to go anywhere, in private house or club, without meeting some gouty man or too stout lady who asserted that a sure cure and preventive for either condition was some drink made with a fresh lemon. It was not surprising, therefore, to find that the chief ingredient in two of the secret remedies first analysed was citric acid.

Bladderwrack (*Fucus vesiculosus*) is a common sea-weed which has earned, it is not quite easy to understand on what grounds, a reputation for reducing corpulency. It contains sodium salts in rather large quantities, and a small proportion of iodine, much less than many other sea-weeds. In Ireland it was once thought to be good for pigs, making them fat, and if it has an opposite effect on human beings, that effect must be very slight and uncertain.

Still, if people like to pay an absurdly high price for citric acid or extract of bladderwrack under other names, it would, perhaps, be churlish to object, but the case is rather different with the extract or other preparation of the thyroid gland found to be present in two of the nostrums most recently analysed. Medical men are not infrequently asked by patients for information or for their opinion with regard to some substance that has been praised in a family newspaper or other easily inspired or corrupted medium to which some authority is ascribed, and the detection of thyroid gland in two of the preparations analysed justifies a note of warning. The administration of thyroid requires to be carefully regulated, and its employment in self-medication cannot be regarded as a safe proceeding. Under these circumstances it can hardly be necessary to say that postal communication with the vendors of the medicines in question, even when accompanied by the patient's answers to printed questions and description of his symptoms, is not only of no value, but may be a source of danger by giving a false sense of security.

It is curious indeed to note that one of these secret preparations, Marmola, does not appear to be advertised to the public as a proprietary article at all, but is named as one ingredient among others in a prescription which is recommended in a paragraph apparently dictated solely by pity for suffering fat people; the chemist to whom the prescription will be taken to be compounded, however, is the recipient of advertising matter urging him to lay in a stock of the article to be in readiness for the demand. It is to be hoped that no chemist would dispense such a " prescription " without making it clear to his customer that what is supplied is a proprietary article, about the usefulness or innocuousness of which he knows nothing; otherwise the customer, who finds it named along with preparations bearing the letters " B.P.," is likely to suppose that it is a known substance, and that the dispensing of the prescription by a chemist indicates that the mixture is a proper and safe one to take. Two of the other preparations described are evidently usually or always supplied to the public without the agency of any retailer, the vendor thus securing the whole profit, which, it will be seen, is considerable. In both these cases the attempt is clearly made to get the customer to pay at once for as large a quantity at possible, presumably because he will be less likely to do so after giving the medicines a trial. The most alluring prospects are, of course, held out in the advertisements, but when the customer has been drawn into correspondence, and especially after he has begun to send his money, a process of " hedging " begins, as will be seen from the extracts quoted from letters sent by the vendors.

Phenolphthalein—a chemical body sold sometimes under the trade names purgen, laxoin, laxatol, laxen, etc.—appears as an ingredient in two of the nostrums, and formamine (hexamethylene-tetramine)—which goes also by many names, urotropine, cystamin, cystogen, metramine, and vesalvine among others—

in one; the preparation containing the latter is said to have been devised as the result of an accident in the laboratory, in which a piece of fat became changed into oil without the rupture of the fat cells, a statement which suggests that the advertiser thinks that fat in the human body is solid like tallow or lard.

ANTIPON.

This preparation is sold by a Company with offices in London. The bottle in which it is sent out holds a little over $6\frac{1}{2}$ fluid ounces and costs 2s. 6d. It bears no label, but has the word "Antipon" blown in the glass. A circular enclosed with the bottle gives a number of rules on the subject of dietary, together with statements as to the merits of the article, from which the following extracts are taken:

As a really permanent cure for corpulence, combining remarkable fat-reducing properties with tonic principles of the highest quality, "Antipon" is justly regarded by the most competent authorities as one of the most valuable discoveries in modern therapeutics, solving once and for all the vexed question of the radical cure of obesity without harmful after-effects. "Antipon" absolutely and definitely replaces all the weakening and frequently dangerous processes, systems and medicines which have hitherto done duty as remedies for the disease of obesity. It provides the medical practitioner and the public with a powerful and entirely harmless specific not hitherto within their reach.

Within a day and a night of taking the first dose there will be a reduction of weight varying from 8 oz. to 3lb., in extreme cases even more. The subsequent daily decrease will be persistent until normal weight and dimensions are attained, when the doses may be discontinued.

Directions for Use.—Take two dessertspoonfuls in half a wineglassful of water, immediately after meals. N.B.—After taking dose, cork the bottle securely.

Analysis showed the liquid to be a solution of citric acid in water, of the strength of 39·3 grains in a fluid ounce; a red colouring substance was also present, and 0·4 per cent. of alcohol, the latter being doubtless introduced with the colouring. The red colour could be perfectly matched with cochineal, but the behaviour towards alkalies and other reagents showed differences; cochineal, with the addition of a little methyl orange, however, showed in most respects a similar behaviour.

The estimated cost of ingredients for $6\frac{1}{2}$ fluid ounces is $1\frac{1}{3}$d.

RUSSELL'S ANTI-CORPULENT PREPARATION.

This preparation is sold from an address in London and like the previous one, was in a bottle bearing no label; the letters "F.C.R." were blown in the glass, and the bottle, which held 12½ fluid ounces and cost 6s., was enclosed in a perfectly plain case, with no printed matter accompanying it. A pamphlet on the subject of the medicine was posted separately to the person ordering it; in this it was explained that:

Acting upon the many suggestions received, principally from ladies, the bottles are packed quite plainly, and without the ordinary trade labels usually found upon medicines, etc. The box is quite devoid of advertisements or anything whatever likely to denote its contents. The servants and others attached to the household may therefore be safely entrusted to open the box; inquisitiveness, if present, will not be rewarded.

In this pamphlet very detailed directions were also given for taking the medicine, and for diet and exercise. It was stated that:

In a very short space of time, say twenty-four hours, a considerable quantity of the most unhealthy fat will have been removed from that part of the system most in need of relief from the adipose matter oppressing it (the quantity varies from 8 oz. to 2 b., or even more).

The dose is one tablespoonful in a half-wineglassful of water, within, say, ten minutes after each meal.

Analysis showed the liquid to consist of a solution of citric acid in water, containing 37 grains in a fluid ounce. The orange colour was found to be due to iron, which was present to the extent of 0·012 per cent.; and 0·4 per cent. of alcohol was also found. Addition of this proportion of iron in the form of the ammonio-citrate was found to give a practically identical colour, and the formula is approximately:

Citric acid	37 grains.
Iron and ammonium citrate	¼ grain.
Rectified spirit	2 minims.
Water	To 1 fluid ounce.

The estimated cost of the ingredients for 12½ fluid ounces is 2·1d.

ABSORBIT REDUCING PASTE AND J. Z. OBESITY TABLETS.

These two preparations are sold by a "Hygienic Skin Specialist." The paste, or, perhaps, both preparations, appear to be also known under the name of "Zobeide," as the paste was supplied in response to an order for "Zobeida," and the jar bore a label giving a so-called "analysis" (which it is needless to say was no analysis) beginning, "We have carefully examined the Zobeide Tissue Absorbers and Paste." The price of the paste was 3s. 6d., and the jar contained just over 2 ounces. The directions on the label were :

> Rub in a circular direction, at night, where needed, for five minutes or more ; firm, even movements, and only use as much as the skin will absorb.

The paste was a pink ointment, containing 93 per cent. of a fatty basis, 4·8 per cent. of a substance which agreed in its characters with dried bile, and was evidently ordinary "purified ox-bile," and a little carmine, the remainder being moisture. Further examination of the fatty basis showed a considerable proportion of beeswax, and the analytical results obtained agreed with a mixture of :

Beeswax	23 parts.
Lard	46 ,,
Rapeseed (colza) oil	31 ,,

It is not possible, however, to assign an exact formula to a mixture of fatty substances like this. The composition of the paste was approximately :

Purified ox bile	5 per cent.
Beeswax	22 ,,
Lard	44 ,,
Oil	29 ,,
Carmine	q.s.

A trace of perfume was also present.

The estimated cost of ingredients (2 ounces) is 3d.
The tablets are sold in boxes, containing 25, price, 2s.
The directions were :

> Two at night dissolved in the mouth as an ordinary lozenge.

The tablets were flat oval lozenges weighing 19 grains each. Analysis showed their composition to be as follows :—

Sulphur	24 per cent.
Ginger, about	4 ,,
Sugar	61 ,,
Acacia gum	8 ,,
Moisture	3 ,,

The estimated cost of the ingredients for 25 lozenges is ½d.

XL REDUCING PILLS AND REDUCING LOTION.

Hughes & Hughes's XL Reducing Pills and Ointment are advertised from an address in a seaside town. The pills are sold in boxes containing 28, price 2s. 9d. a box. The preparation was described, in a circular enclosed with the box, as:

> A remedy at once safe, speedy, and efficacious, and of marked value from the health point of view, as it combats the special ills to which the corpulent have a liability. It is very easy to take, the pills being tasteless, and does not necessarily oblige any special course of diet.

The directions were:

> 2 pills, twice a day, after principal meals.

The pills were coated with French chalk, and coloured pink on the outside. After removal of the coating they had an average weight of 3 grains. Analysis showed them to contain a vegetable extract, powdered ginger, powdered liquorice, iron, potassium, phosphate, and iodide; in addition to the mineral constituents just named, the ash showed all the constituents of the ash of extract of bladderwrack; various other tests applied to the pills indicated this extract to be present, and failed to show any other ingredients. The quantities of the respective substances were determined as accurately as possible, and the formula found to be approximately:

Potassium iodide	0·15 grain.
Iron phosphate	0·35 ,,
Powdered ginger	0·2 ,,
,, liquorice	0·1 ,,
Extract of *Fucus vesiculosus*	2·2 grains.
In one pill.	

The estimated cost of the ingredients for 28 pills is 1¼d.

The Reducing Lotion for external use only with the XL reducing Pills is sold at 4s. 6d. a bottle, containing 2¼ fluid ounces.

> Directions for Use.—To a little of the lotion add three or four times the amount of water (to a spoonful, three or four spoonfuls of water). The lotion is in a highly-concentrated form, and equals a bottle four times the size. The lotion should be applied night and morning, gently, without rubbing, by means of the hand, or a piece of rag, to the part desired. Any part that is abnormally enlarged can be so treated, except the face, to which it should not be applied. The XL lotion will not irritate the most delicate skin, but it should not be used when there is any scratch or abrasion.

Analysis showed the presence of chloride, bromide, and iodide of potassium, glycerine, and a small quantity of a resinous substance in combination with alkali. The amount of the last constituent was very small, the resinous substance only amounting to 0·08 per cent.; it was somewhat bitter, with little colour, and showed no characteristic reactions or properties by which it could be identified. The proportions of the other ingredients were found to be :

Potassium iodide	....	9·7 grains.
,, bromide....	....	13·5 ,,
,, chloride....	....	6·9 ,,
Glycerine	....	105 minims.
Water....	....	To 1 fluid ounce.

The estimated cost of the ingredients (2¼ fluid ounces) is about ¾d.

TRILENE TABLETS.

These tablets are advertised from an address in London, in boxes price 2s. 6d., containing 66 tablets.

Enclosed with the package was a little book containing testimonials, directions, etc., and also a small circular giving instructions as to diet, with the addition :

We desire to say that such precautions are not indispensable by any means, but we formulate the above for the guidance of those in whom any peculiarity of Constitution may render such care salutary, and to promote rapidity of cure.

The directions were :

Three of the tablets three times a day 10 minutes before meals, either dissolved on the tongue or taken as pills. (*No change of diet being essential.*)

It was also added :

The present supply lasts one week, in which time the weight begins to lessen, but a marked change in appearance naturally occupies *several weeks* to effect.

Two separate packages of the tablets were obtained for analysis at an interval of several weeks ; in the first supply the tablets were of a dirty white colour and contained no dye, but in the second they were bright yellow, and contained a yellow dye, which appeared to be one of the coal-tar colours ; the other ingredients were the same as those found on the first occasion. The average weight of one tablet was 0·9 grain, and they were found to contain 87 per cent. of sugar, 2·4 per cent. of moisture, and 0·5 per cent. of ash ; about three-quarters of the remainder was starch, principally potato starch, but with a little maize. The residual 2 or 3 per cent. was a gelatinous substance which showed no marked reactions or characters, and exhibited only traces of cell tissue when examined microscopically. Analysis of the ash showed it to contain sodium, potassium, calcium and magnesium chloride, sulphate, and phosphate; these are the constant constituents of the ash of extract of *Fucus vesiculosus*; an aqueous extract of the tablets contained a small quantity of mucilage similar to that yielded by the same drug. By taking some *Fucus vesiculosus* in the wet state, pounding it to a pulp and boiling it, a material was obtained agreeing with the gelatinous substance from the tablets, and there appeared no ground for doubting the identity of the two. Careful search was made for alkaloids and other substances in small quantity, but without any being found. The formula thus became:

Fucus vesiculosus, in pulp	3 per cent. (dry weight).
Starch	7 ,,
Sugar	87 ,,
Water	3 ,,
Yellow dye	q.s.

The estimated cost of the ingredients (66 tablets) is one-fortieth of a penny.

HARGREAVE'S REDUCING WAFERS.

This preparation is supplied from an address in London in boxes price 1s. 1½d., containing 21.

The following extracts are taken from a circular enclosed with the box; the circular contained also a number of testimonials, with directions, etc.

Purely vegetable. Contain nothing harmful. Can be taken at any time with perfect safety. Dose: Three wafers daily. One after Breakfast, Dinner and Supper. If Supper is not taken, one after Tea instead. May be dissolved on the tongue or taken as pills. No change in diet necessary.

The supply sent herewith lasts one week, in which time the Fat commences to get less. In most cases, however, to complete a cure takes about seven weeks, therefore clients should now send for the further six weeks' treatment.

The "wafers" were really compressed tablets of the ordinary shape, coated with French chalk, and coloured pink externally with eosin. After removing the coating the average weight of the tablets was 2·4 grains; they consisted of substances of "extract" nature, with about 10 per cent. of powdered liquorice. Analysis of the ash showed all the constituents of the ash of extract of *Fucus vesiculosus*

(bladderwrack), and other tests indicated that this extract formed about one-half of the tablet; the other constituent (or constituents) also of "extract" nature, showed no reactions or properties by which it could be identified, and it was probably present merely as excipient.

ALLAN'S ANTI-FAT.

This substance is supplied by an American "Botanic Medicine Company" from a London office, in bottles containing 6½ fluid ounces, price 6s. 6d.

On the wrapper appeared the words:

Purely vegetable. Perfectly harmless. Always efficacious.

We call special attention to the efficacy of our Anti-Fat in the cure of that distressing complaint—indigestion or dyspepsia. It acts solely upon the food in the stomach, regulating and putting the liver and discharging organs in good working order.

A circular was enclosed with the bottle, entitled, "How to get lean without starvation," from which the following extracts are taken:

A very extensive observation has convinced us, since our first circular treatise was issued, that in the majority of cases the Anti-Fat must be taken for from two to three, and, in rare cases, even four weeks before the patient will begin to notice much reduction of flesh, after which the loss goes on rapidly—generally from three to five pounds a week. In some cases the diminution in weight commences from the first two or three days' use of it.

The treatment of obesity has hitherto rested on no sure basis.

Through the study of physiological chemistry, a *specific* has at length been discovered, which, from the name of the discoverer, has been called Allan's Anti-Fat.

Directions: Take two teaspoonfuls of the Anti-Fat in a wineglass full of water or sweet milk before each meal.

A small slip was also enclosed headed "CAUTION!!" which stated:

The color, as well as the flavor, of the Anti-Fat, varies somewhat with age and exposure to light, but neither in the least impairs its virtues. The temperature of the weather at the time of the manufacture of this remedy has also much to do with its clearness, or transparency, but does not affect its properties.

Analysis showed the presence of alcohol, glycerine, potassium iodide, salicylic acid, and a vegetable extract which from its properties and the analysis of the ash was evidently a purified extract of *Fucus vesiculosus*. The proportion of the latter drug represented could not, of course, be determined with certainty for the reasons already given, but the amounts of the other ingredients were ascertained by analysis, and the formula was approximately as follows:

Potassium iodide	0·3 grain.
Salicylic acid	1·0 ,,
Glycerine	40 minims.
Fluid extract of *Fucus vesiculosus*	70 ,,
Water	To 1 fluid ounce.

The estimated cost of the ingredients (6½ fluid ounces) is 3d.

MARMOLA.

This preparation is supplied by another American Company, which also has a depôt in London. It is sold in packages, containing ½ ounce, price 2s. 6d.

This preparation, which has been largely advertised in daily and weekly newspapers, is not represented as a proprietary article, but is mentioned as one ingredient of a prescription to be made up at a chemist's. The following advertisement is a sample:

Is Fatness a Social Offence ?

"The female form, being capable of expressing a supreme degree of grace, should be an inspiration in our daily lives and lead up to higher ideals of beauty," said an art lecturer lately. Therefore the fat woman is an enemy to the artistic uplift, for she is entirely too heavy for any wings of fancy to raise.

Why should any woman remain fat when it is so easy to reduce one's flesh ? A woman may take but little exercise and enjoy the best of food, and still preserve a beautiful figure. She has at hand a simple fat-reducer that takes the place of starving and gymnastics. It consists of a dessertspoonful after meals and at bedtime of this simple mixture: One half-ounce of Marmola, one ounce of fluid extract of Glycyrrhiza B.P., one ounce of pure Glycerine B.P., and Peppermint Water to make six ounces in all. Every over-fat person should try it. It's quite harmless, and will take off as much as a pound of fat a day. With a chemist's handy, anyone can have a good figure at a reasonable cost.

A dessertspoonful of the mixture prescribed would contain about 9 or 10 grains of Marmola. The prescription and directions were reproduced on the label of the package, and it was added:

If faithfully taken as directed for 60 or 90 days, satisfactory results should be obtained.

which is a decidedly milder statement than that in the advertisement that it " will take off as much as a pound of fat a day."

The box contained a light brown powder, and analysis showed the presence of (1) a large proportion of a powdered seaweed, agreeing well in characters with the powder of *Fucus vesiculosus*, its identity being further indicated by the composition of the ash; (2) a substance of proteid nature, agreeing well in characters with the powder of dried thyroid gland, its identity being further indicated by the presence of iodine in organic combination; (3) phenolphthalein; (4) sodium chloride (common salt); and (5) extractive. The last showed no well-marked characters by which it could be identified, and differed both in quantity and some minor properties from the extracts obtained from a specimen of powdered fucus which was used for comparison. This difference might quite well be due to differences in the drug or in the treatment it had received, or the extract may represent some other ingredient possessed of no distinctive characters; a trace of oil of peppermint was also present.

Although it was easy to ascertain the nature of the ingredients the determination of the proportions in which they were present in such a mixture offered no little difficulty. It is not necessary to detail here the methods employed, but it will suffice to say that while every care was taken to make the results as accurate as possible, they cannot in the nature of the case be more than approximate. The formula arrived at was:

		In one Dose.
Dried thyroid gland....	14 per cent.	1·4 grain.
Phenolphthalein	4 ,,	0·4 ,,
Sodium chloride	7 ,,	0·7 ,,
Powdered *Fuscus vesiculosus*	50 ,,	5·0 grains.
Extractive....	25 ,,	2·5 ,,
Oil of peppermint	trace	trace.

Taking the "extractive" at the price of some of the commoner medicinal extracts, the estimated cost of the ingredients for half an ounce is about 4d.

FIGUROIDS.

The tablets sold under the name of Figuroids are or were recently supplied by a London Company, price 2s. 9d. per bottle, containing 12 large and 12 small tablets.

They were described in a pamphlet enclosed in the package as

A Scientific Obesity Cure discovered through an accident while making Scientific Investigations in the Laboratory.

Other extracts from the pamphlet are as follows:

In looking through quantities of anti-fat literature one finds all kinds of crude, ignorant explanations, such as, for example, that the remedy absorbs the fat. Now, a sponge absorbs water, or any dry thing will absorb a liquid, but common sense will tell you that a liquid taken into the body will not absorb fat; you can clearly understand that point without further explanation. Another remedy, it is claimed, simply destroys the fat. This explanation is, as you can see, equally preposterous. In Nature nothing is destroyed. When a piece of coal is burned it is not destroyed, it is only changed into gases and smoke, and fat is not destroyed by any remedy.

Now here is the true and scientific explanation. When Figuroids are taken, and the fat passes out of those cells into the circulation, it is oxidized. This produces chiefly water and carbonic acid gas. This oxidation takes place while it is being carried along in the circulating blood. This carbonic acid gas and water vapour are eliminated from the system as already explained.

When you take Figuroids, therefore, your extra fat simply passes from the adipose cells through their unbroken walls into the blood, and is there changed to water and Carbon Dioxide, and thus leaves the body.

This is the scientific, simple, natural explanation, and Figuroids is the only remedy which has the effect. . . .

If then you are exceedingly stout and suffering from all the unpleasant symptoms resulting from that condition, if you find your weight excessive, if you suffer from heart palpitation, if you have redness of the face with annoying perspiration and shiny appearance of the nose and face, if the throat and bosom are altogether too stout, and if the lines of the figure have been lost, or if the abdomen has become too prominent, if Gout and Rheumatism make themselves manifest occasionally, and all the disagreeable and often dangerous symptoms of Obesity are apparent, you will know that in Figuroids you have a perfectly safe remedy, while if you suffer but slightly from Obesity and all the symptoms are less marked, you will also know that Figuroids furnish you with an effective, agreeable, and perfectly Safe cure. . . .

When taking Figuroids it is not necessary to unduly restrict yourself in the matter of diet. You may eat and drink what you desire in reason. It would of course, be foolish to drink or eat excessively of fat or fattening foods.

In another enclosed circular the Company stated that:

They have decided to originate a No Cure No Payment system, and will refund the purchase money to any patient whose weight is not reduced by from two to six pounds per month whilst taking Figuroids. . . . This offer to refund purchase money is made on the understanding that the Figuroid Company's instructions are faithfully observed and the conditions of their offer compled with.

The directions on the label were as follows:

Each bottle contains an equal number of full doses (large tablet) and half doses (small tablet).

Take regularly one full dose (large tablet) dissolved in plain or soda water within 30 minutes after each of the first three meals on the first day. Next day take one half dose (small tablet) dissolved in plain or soda water within 30 minutes after each of the three meals. Third day take full doses again; and so continue alternating.

Although it is here clearly conveyed, without directly making the statement, that the large and small tablets only differ in being full doses and half doses respectively, examination showed their composition to be different, and it was necessary to analyse them separately.

Large Tablets.

The large tablets had an average weight of 58 grains; analysis showed them to contain an effervescing mixture of sodium bicarbonate and tartaric acid, in which the former was in excess, so that the resulting product was alkaline, together with sodium chloride (common salt), phenolphthalein, formamine (hexamethylene-tetramine), talc, and gum. The quantity of each of the ingredients was determined as accurately as possible, with the results given below; it will be noted that these quantities add up to 101·4 instead of 100, the reason being that the whole of the soda is for convenience represented as bicarbonate, whereas a portion of it had become converted to carbonate by loss of carbon dioxide.

		In One Tablet.
Sodium bicarbonate....	62·0 per cent.	38·9 grains.
Tartaric acid....	22·6 ,,	13·1 ,,
Sodium chloride	6·5 ,,	3·8 ,,
Phenolphthalein	2·0 ,,	1·2 ,,
Formamine	3·5 ,,	2·0 ,,
Talc	2·8 ,,	
Gum about	2·0 ,,	

Hexamethylene-tetramine or formamine, is perhaps better known by its trade names—urotropine, cystamin, urisol, etc.; it does not appear to have been described as of value for obesity.

Small Tablets.

The small tablets had an average weight of 34·3 grains. Analysis showed them to contain sodium bicarbonate and tartaric acid, but in this case the latter was in excess and the product acid; the other ingredients were sodium chloride, phenolphthalein, and talc. The results of quantitative determinations indicated the following formula (more carbon dioxide had been lost in this case; the figures add up to 108·5, the reason being that given above):

		In One Tablet.
Sodium bicarbonate....	34·8 per cent.	11·9 grains.
Tartaric acid....	46·3 ,,	15·9 ,,
Sodium chloride	22·8 ,,	7·6 ,,
Phenolphthalein	1·6 ,,	0·5 grain.
Talc	3·0 ,,	

The estimated cost of the ingredients of the contents of a 2s. 9d. bottle is 1¾d.

FELL REDUCING TREATMENT.

In pushing this "treatment," advertised by an Association giving an address in London, the system of letters in series is resorted to, but a small package, containing 112 tablets, can be purchased for 6s. 6d.

An advertisement ran as follows:

FAT PEOPLE GIVEN FREE TREATMENT.

We have such marvellous records of reductions effected in hundreds of cases with the Fell Reducing Treatment, that we have decided, for a limited period only, to give free trial treatments.

7 LB. PER WEEK REDUCTION IS GUARANTEED, without dieting. Perfectly harmless, pleasant; easy and quick results. Send no money. Simply address the Fell Formula Association, 340, Century House, 205, Regent Street, London, W., enclosing stamp to pay postage, when a free supply in plain wrapper will be immediately forwarded.

A free supply was sent on application, accompanied by a letter and sundry circulars; other letters followed at intervals, and extracts from some of these will be given. They were printed in imitation of typewriting, with the name and address typed in, so as to give the appearance of being personal letters. It will be noted that when a customer has been attracted by the advertisement that "7 lb. per week reduction is guaranteed, without dieting," very much smaller claims are gradually substituted.

Esteemed Friend,
   Your favour of recent date has received our careful attention, and we take pleasure in sending you a three days' trial of the Fell Reducing Treatment. Before taking it, weigh yourself, and then again in three days, on the same scales and in the same clothes, you will find you have lost some 3 lb. in weight.

An abnormal condition like corpulency requires that the antidote directly reaches the seat of the complaint, and by these Reducers the blood will be purified, and all the organs of the body restored to natural healthy action, while the germs of the disease will be entirely eradicated from the system, so that the superfluous fat, which will be removed will not return. . . .

At the present stage of the disease in your case, we can positively assure you that under our treatment a marked improvement will begin at once, and continue steadily until a complete reduction in weight, with all the benefits to general health, is effected. Unlike most other methods of treatment, the action begins immediately and the sufferer feels better almost from the beginning, and it is with confidence that we advise you to begin a course of treatment with our Reducing Preparation at once.

Our regular terms and prices are 26s. for a case containing three 11s. boxes, whereby a saving of 7s. is effected.

If you take up the treatment in this manner you can be sure of having sufficient of the Tablets to take you through to a quick reduction. Single boxes of Tablets, however, are supplied at 11s. and smaller sizes at 6s. 6d. The 6s. 6d. box covers a ten days' treatment, while the 11s. boxes contain three times the quantity of the 6s. 6d.

This letter was not answered, but before long another was received which contained the following passages :

In sending you the sample of the " Fell " Preparation, we did so more to show the thorough nature of our treatment than from the expectation that material benefit would be realized from same. As you require to bring about a certain reduction you must necessarily undergo a certain course of treatment. A pound a day reduction results in many cases, and there is every reason to expect that such reduction can be effected in yours. A serious affliction such as obesity is not to be removed by any temporary remedy or with a few days' treatment. . . .

Remember, a 26s. case contains sufficient treatment to reduce materially the most stubborn and long-standing case, while an 11s. box contains three times the quantity of the 6s. 6d. box. . . .

A supply was sent for and was accompanied by the following letter :

Dear Sir,

I have despatched to you the Tablets together with directions and instructions. I ask you to carefully observe same, and am confident if you do so, you will very soon see most beneficial results. . . .

I am confident that you will be highly delighted with the splendid effects of the Tablets at the end of a few weeks if you follow carefully my instructions and are prompt and regular in taking the Tablets. I am sending you herewith printed instructions and rules for diet. You will note that our suggestion as to what you should eat, if strictly followed, will not work any hardship, and that you will never go hungry. . . .

This letter, signed "————' Adviser, Fell Formula Association,'" was accompanied by a printed circular giving rules as to diet, etc., and by a "symptom blank," to be filled up by the patient in order to obtain particulars of "the Fell System of Simple Muscular Movements for Reducing the Weight and Increasing the Strength, in combination with the 'Fell' Reducing Treatment"; it appears from the latter that particulars of these exercises are only supplied when the 26s. case is sent for.

A fourth letter dealt with generalities and recommended taking the reducing treatment in increased quantities, but after an interval a fifth was received, enclosing a booklet advocating the use of "the Century Thermal Bath Cabinet," from which the following are extracts:

. . . We have strongly recommended the Home Turkish Bath that it may be used at least once a week as an adjunct to the Reducing Treatment; hence our affiliation to the "Century Thermal" Bath Cabinet, Ltd., whose home cabinet is built on such lines as to render it the best device extant for taking Hot Air or Vapour Baths.

. . . in any event, it were better to spend the required amount, for were the cost as much as £10 in all (it has but rarely exceeded that) the expense is out of all proportion to the ultimate benefit.

. . . with the Fell treatment no case of obesity, in either sex, can fail to be reduced if assisted with the regular use of the Hot Air Bath.

Booklets entitled *Corpulence or Obesity. Its causes, results, and successful treatment: The Treatment of Obesity by the " Fell" Reducing Treatment:* and *Make Muscle of your Fat*, were also sent at different times. The following extracts from two of these scarcely appear consistent:

A Guarantee to Reduce Weight.

It is not our purpose to indulge in empty talk only, or in unconsequential boasts. We are prepared to, and do, give a positive guarantee that the Fell Treatment, used in conjunction with the Muscular System, will reduce the fat of any person—provided our instructions are adhered to—in the space of a very few weeks.

Do We Guarantee ?

We are frequently asked this question personally and by letter, and reply emphatically—No, we do not. To say Yes—would be illogical and certainly demoralising.

A guarantee that any medical remedy or curative will absolutely effect its stated purpose is misleading, deceptive, delusive, and is a trap to ensnare, not intelligent individuals, but the unwary, the unsophisticated, and those utterly unable to discriminate as to the merits or demerits of any so-called specific.

The dose was stated to be :

Nine tablets daily. Three taken three times a day before meals. They may be taken as pills or dissolved on the tongue.

The tablets had an average weight of 1 grain. Analysis showed them to contain 90·8 per cent. of milk sugar, 2·4 per cent. of greasy matter, which appeared to be a mixture of stearic acid and paraffin, evidently employed as a lubricant in making the tablets, and 6·8 per cent. of an extract which agreed well in its characters with extract of *Fucus vesiculosus ;* its identity was further indicated by analysis of the ash. Each tablet would thus contain :

Extract of bladderwrack	0·07 grain.
Milk sugar	0·91 ,,

The estimated cost of the ingredients for 112 tablets is ¼d.

NELSON LLOYD SAFE REDUCING TREATMENT.

In this instance the bait of free trial for a fortnight is held out in the advertisements issued from an address in London ; the following are extracts from one advertisement :

I myself am a member of a family many of whom died prematurely after much mental and physical suffering, arising from corpulence. While studying medicine for my degree, I saw the signs of the family complaint in myself. I naturally sought to avert what I for some time feared as being my hereditary fate. It was when I had almost given up hope that I discovered a cure for my condition, which all the time grew worse, in spite of my hopeful trials of all advertised and unadvertised remedies for stoutness. I at last gave up expecting a cure from other people. I experimented with my own thought-out remedies, and, happily, at last my perseverance—or, rather, my desperation—succeeded. . : :

The result of several years' study and experience has only served to make my treatment more and more successful. ∎ ∎ ∎

I specially invite those who have tried other remedies for reducing weight without success to write me for :

I. A copy of my book, " The Scientific Treatment of Obesity " (just published, price 6d.), thoroughly deals with the subject in a popular, readable style. . . .

II. Two photos of the lady referred to above, with her letter giving full particulars of her cure.

III. Everything required for a complete fourteen days' free trial treatment.

I make no charge for all the above, but ask you to enclose sixpence (by postal order), just to cover the expenses of carriage, packing, and dispatch of parcel.

Application for the " Treatment " brought a box containing 42 tablets, a copy of the booklet mentioned above, and a letter and form for particulars. A few extracts will suffice to show what was claimed and the methods adopted.

From the booklet:

Different cases vary so much that the same treatment is never exactly suited to any two cases. Moreover, the treatment has to be modified as the patient progresses, the condition of the individual being periodically allowed for. . . . I wish to make it perfectly clear that not only do I offer every client the full benefit of practically a life study of the whole subject of corpulence, but that I *guarantee* to effect a cure of every case I take up.

There are no "ifs" and "buts" about my promises to my patients. I undertake to reduce corpulence by rational individual treatment in each and every case entrusted to me, and I undertake to promise (*sic*) that my treatment is in no way weakening, that it is permanent, and also that it has absolutely no ill effects.

From the first letter:

One of the Tablets should be taken after each of the three chief meals of the day for the next fortnight. I suggest that if convenient you weigh yourself before beginning the course, and again in fourteen days' time, with the same scales and in the same clothes. You will find you have lost weight, while improving in your general condition. . . . My course of Treatment lasts a month except in unusual cases. The tablets I have sent you for the first fortnight will at once put a stop to the fat-forming habit of the body; these tablets are taken during the first fortnight in all cases, and while excellent results follow even in this brief period, they need to be followed up from the fifteenth day by additional and different remedies, adapted to each individual case.

In order to prepare this part of your Treatment I shall need to have before me full particulars of your case, which you can easily give me by filling up the Consultation Form enclosed herewith. . . . . .

My fee for a month's course of Treatment is one guinea, but you will see that I have given you credit for the first fortnight's Treatment sent you herewith, because this is free in accordance with my offer through the Press. This means that by sending at once you can have one month's complete treatment for half cost. To secure this concession you must, however, send me the Consultation Form filled up, and remittance for 10s. 6d. in time to continue your Treatment on the fifteenth day, and I must have at least three clear days in which to consider your case and prepare and post your Treatment to reach you in time.

The "Consultation Form" contained questions as to age, height, weight, chest and abdomen measurements, details of bodily condition, habits, and diet; this was filled up so as to represent an ordinary case of moderate obesity, and returned with 10s. 6d. In the next letter it was stated:

I am preparing your second fortnight's treatment, and it will be forwarded in due course, but I feel I should like to take this opportunity of pointing out to you that there are special features about your case which, while not preventing the accomplishment of the improvement you desire, will, however, entail a little longer course of treatment than one month.

In my opinion your case requires a two months' course of my treatment, at the end of which time the results will be all that you can desire. I thought it only right you should know this, and I would like you to tell me if you will take the full course my experience leads me to advise you.

My fee for the two months' course is two guineas, but you have already standing to your credit the sum of one guinea, being one half-guinea allowed for first fortnight's free trial, and the other half-guinea you have just sent me.

I should like you to take the full course my experience tells me is necessary for you, and if you now send me the one guinea balance, I will at once arrange for the supply of all the necessary remedies to you at the proper intervals.

The second fortnight's treatment consisted of "special tablets" and a liquid; these were accompanied by a further letter, a diet table, and a report form, to be filled in and returned after 10 days.

The three kinds of medicine were examined with results as follows:

The preliminary tablets.—There were 42 in the box, and the directions were to take one three times a day after meals.

They were sugar-coated and coloured red externally; after removal of the coating, they had an average weight of 4·7 grains. Analysis showed them to consist principally of substances of extract nature, together with an amount of liquorice fibre representing about 20 per cent. of powdered liquorice; iodine was present in organic combination, and a nitrogenous substance; the amount of nitrogen was 0·51 per cent., representing 3·2 per cent. of proteid; no tissue of thyroid gland was present, and the nitrogenous material was probably contained in an extract of this substance. The remainder possessed the general characters of extract of *Fucus vesiculosus*, and its identity was also indicated by analysis of the ash; some gum was also present, and some indication was obtained of another substance also, which, however, possessed no important characters, and was probably also of the nature of excipient. The formula indicated by the results was thus:

Extract of bladderwrack	2·5 grains.
Proteid of thyroid gland	0·15 grain.
Powdered liquorice	0·9 ,,
Excipient and moisture, etc.	q.s. |// In one tablet.

The "special" tablets.—There were 33 of these in a box; the directions were to take one after the mid-day and one after the evening meal. They were sugar-coated but not coloured. After removal of the coating, they had an average weight of 4·6 grains. Analysis showed their composition to agree qualitatively with that of the preliminary tablets, but the nitrogenous material and the liquorice were present in somewhat larger amounts. The following formula was indicated by the results:

Extract of bladderwrack	2·5 grains.
Proteid of thyroid gland	0·19 grain.
Powdered liquorice	1·4 ,,
Excipient and moisture, etc.	q.s.

In one tablet.

The liquid.—Two fluid ounces were supplied, the directions being to take 30 drops in a wineglassful of cold water the last thing at night before retiring and on rising in the morning. Analysis showed this to contain alcohol, glycerine, nitrogenous matter, a little iodine in organic combination, and substances of extract nature; the character of the extract and the composition of the ash again pointed to its being derived from *Fucus vesiculosus;* the amount of nitrogen was determined and the equivalent amount of proteid matter calculated; the alcohol and glycerine were also determined quantitatively; the amount of extract of bladderwrack could only be arrived at by difference, supported by the probability that the alcohol was all, or nearly all, added in the form of the fluid extract of this drug, and the figure can therefore only be given with reservation; there were also indications of some small amount of flavouring and colouring matter having been added. The approximate formula appeared to be:

Proteid of thyroid gland	0·3 part.
Liquid extract of bladderwrack	32 fluid parts.
Glycerine	12 ,,

In 100 fluid parts.

The amount of thyroid actually represented by the nitrogenous matter found in these three preparations was too uncertain for an estimate of the cost price to be of value.

CORPULIN, AND DALLOFF'S TEA "CONTRE L'OBESITÉ" GRAZIANA ZEHRKUR.

Of the German preparations examined by Dr. Zernik two contain bladderwrack. One called Corpulin contains also tamarind and cascara sagrada. The other, Dalloff's Tea "Contre l'Obesité," as to which the advertisers assert that " regular use leads to the removal of superfluous adipose tissue and the person becomes healthy and attains old age" was found to consist of a mixture of the leaves of senna, bearberry (*Uvæ ursi*) and lavender, and anthylla flowers. Any action it may have depends probably on the senna leaves. It is sold in boxes costing 7s. 6d. or 4s. 6d. ; the smaller box contains 80 grammes, or nearly 3 ounces of the powder.

Graziana Reducing Treatment (Zehrkur) is sent out in parcels costing 3s. Each contains a packet of a greyish-brown powder, a box of 40 starch capsules, each containing $0\cdot 2$ gramme of a light brown finely-divided powder, and a box of 86 pills, each weighing $0\cdot 22$ gramme. The chief ingredient of each of the preparations is powdered *Fucus*. The pills contain some substance yielding emodin, the purgative principle, or one of the purgative principles, of aloes, rhubarb, buckthorn, and senna, and also some sulphates and chlorides.

CHAPTER X.

SKIN DISEASES.

PROPRIETARY articles for the cure of eczema and other skin affections include several which are as widely advertised as any nostrums of any kind. Some of them are at first offered at the comparatively low price of 1s. 1½d.; but in almost every case the further information supplied on application shows that what is really recommended is a "treatment," including an ointment or other application, a special soap, and a medicine to be taken internally, and often also a dusting powder, and occasionally other articles. The importance of persisting in the treatment is strongly emphasised, with the result that anyone who once lays out 1s. 1½d. is likely to be drawn into spending quite a considerable sum. Only a few out of the long list which might be made of these articles have been analysed, but the results throw sufficient light on the general nature of the whole class. The most striking point about them is perhaps the extremely commonplace nature of the drugs selected, although the vendors in some instances would have the buyer believe that the preparation sold is the result of years of patient experiment.

ANTEXEMA.

A Company with an address in London advertises for sale a bottle, price 1s. 1½d., containing a little less than 1½ ounces, but the "Antexema Treatment" includes Antexema, Antexema Soap, and Antexema Granules (to be taken internally). On a handbill enclosed with the bottle it was stated that:

> In most cases " Antexema " will by itself effect a cure, but the permanence of this is assured by the continued use of a suitable soap, and the cleansing and purifying action of " Antexema Granules " on the blood.

A booklet on "Skin Troubles" was also enclosed, containing some "before" and "after" illustrations, but they could hardly be expected to convince anyone; directions were given in this for the course to be pursued in a variety of disorders, including such "skin troubles" as in-growing toenails, lupus, piles, ulcers, etc. Incidentally, twelve other preparations made by the same Company, in addition to the three named above, were recommended.

On the outer package it was stated that :

"Antexema" is the most efficacious remedy known for the relief of all inflamed conditions of the skin. Its beneficial effects are not confined to the curing of Eczema, Psoriasis, Nettlerash, Erysipelas, Boils, and other serious troubles, but it is also by far the best remedy for Cuts, Burns, Sores, Bruises, Chilblains, Blisters, Insect bites, and every variety of trouble to which the skin is liable.

Only "Antexema" itself was analysed. It consisted of an emulsion, with more or less of a watery layer below it. The directions for use were :

Shake the bottle well, and, if necessary, stir up the contents until a milky substance is formed. Then gently rub "Antexema" into the parts affected until dry, and if the case is a severe one it should be applied as often as possible. "Antexema" is odourless, non-poisonous, and invisible when rubbed on the skin, and it instantly allays irritation. Do not wash any weeping or inflamed surface until healed, and, if possible, avoid dressings and coverings.

Analysis showed it to consist of :

Soft paraffin	35·4 per cent.
Boric acid	1·5 ,,
Gummy matter	12·4 ,,
Water	50·7 ,,

The gum resembled in some respects a mixture of acacia and tragacanth, but could not be exactly identified.

The estimated cost of the ingredients of 1½ ounces is two-thirds of a penny.

PACIDERMA PREPARATIONS.

These preparations are advertised as follows from an address in London :

New Cure for Eczema.—A victim who was cured after 5 years' intense suffering will gladly send to all readers of the *Christian Herald* full particulars (free) of an inexpensive guaranteed cure for Eczema, Bad Legs, Sore Hands and all Skin Eruptions, on receipt of stamped addressed envelope.—Write to A. Paciderma.

An application to the address given brought a typed letter apparently produced on a multiple copy machine, from "Paciderma. Manageress, Mrs. E. Avice," from which the following extracts are taken :

"Paciderma" .... consists of three preparations (in one package), one for internal use and two for external use. Both internal and external Remedies are absolutely necessary to eradicate the disease. . . . The price is most moderate, namely 6s. and postage 3d. for the package containing the three preparations for thirty days' full treatment. In conclusion I would point out to you that these Remedies have met with a world-wide success, even in the worst forms of these terrible complaints, and are in fact so wonderfully successful that they are
GUARANTEED EFFICACIOUS IN EVERY CASE
no matter what has previously been tried and failed. . . . Be sure to fill up the Order Form which I am enclosing you as carefully and accurately as you can so that I may be able to give your case my fullest attention and consideration.

This letter was accompanied by a booklet entitled "Eczema and how to Cure it," and by an order form with spaces for name, address, date, and the following further particulars :

Age ; sex ; occupation ; how long been suffering ? where the complaint is located ; are the spots or wounds dry ? is there any sticky discharge ? are your bowels constipated ? do you suffer from piles ? do you suffer from indigestion ? do you suffer from rheumatism or gout ? Do you suffer from any other complaint ?

This form, filled up with the details of an imaginary case, was sent with a postal order for the requisite amount. A case of "Paciderma" preparations was at once received, and needless to say there was no evidence of their having been modified in any way in consequence of the " fullest attention and consideration " given to the particulars supplied. The preparations were accompanied by a further letter, typed like the first, from which the following is extracted :

One case of the remedies is generally sufficient to effect a cure, and I trust that it may be so in your case, but if the disease has been in the system for years it has got a firm hold, and naturally takes longer to eradicate ; therefore, if this case of remedies should not cure you, you must lose no time in writing for a further supply so that no time may be lost between. You must avoid anything likely to irritate the skin, and be especially careful as to the soap you use, as many soaps are most injurious, being quite sufficient in themselves to cause an eruption. I should recommend you to use " Paciderma Skin Soap " to wash yourself with, as it is absolutely pure, and will keep your skin smooth and healthy.

After an interval a further letter was received, which ran as follows :

Dear Sir,—I have been expecting to hear from you as to how the treatment I sent you some time ago has affected you. I sincerely trust that you have derived benefit from it. As I think I told you before, some cases are naturally much more difficult to cure than others, and take longer time, as in most cases the disease has been for years getting a firm hold on the system, and cannot, therefore, be eradicated in a few days.

I assure you I should be the last to induce you to spend money, unless I honestly thought and believed that the treatment would benefit you. I have been a fellow sufferer myself, and know what it did for me by persevering after everything else had failed. If, therefore, you are not yet cured, I think it is only my duty to strongly urge you to persevere with the treatment, and if you hesitate to do so owing to the money being a consideration to you, I am willing to meet you as far as I possibly can, and will send you the complete 6s. 3d. case for 4s. 6d. post free, which is just cost price, or I will send you the Blood Wafers for 2s. 2d. per box post free instead of 2s. 10d., or the Crème for 2s. 2d. post free instead of 2s. 10d., or the Powder for 7d. instead of 9d. post free.

I am offering you this very great reduction in price as I am most anxious that you should be cured, as I am quite certain that you will be if you persevere steadily.

Do not be afraid of troubling me by writing me fully as to how the treatment has affected you, as I can assure you that I am quite as anxious to cure you as you yourself are to be cured, and I take a special interest in your case.

Trusting soon to hear from you,

Yours truly,

E. AVICE.

The booklet already referred to contained a sworn statement by Mrs. Avice detailing her own sufferings and cure, the latter being due to " a dear old friend, an M.D." Further paragraphs, not in the sworn statement, were as follows :

It remained for my old friend, the Doctor, to whose discoveries I owe my cure, to find the only certain remedy for this dread complaint. For years he studied and searched to find a cure for that curse of hot climates, the " prickly heat," a very distressing form of Eczema which is very prevalent in warm countries, and which few Europeans escape. At last his perseverance was rewarded, and the long sought for Remedy found and used with the greatest success both abroad and after his return to England. Since his death I have still further improved on and perfected his ideas, and have evolved my now well-known " Paciderma," which has met with the most startling success in every case in which it has been tried. . . .

Paciderma cures all skin troubles without exception, all pimples, blotches, sores and eruptions of every kind, in sufferers of every age, from the infant at the breast to the old and infirm man or woman who has reached or passed the allotted span of three score years and ten.

It is absolutely the only cure for Eczema.

The following are the results of the examination of the remedies evolved after so much study and research and perfected and improved :

Paciderma Crème.—Price 2s. 9d. per box, holding nearly 4 ounces. Directions for use :

Apply the Crème to the parts affected with the finger, or spread on lint or soft linen, and bandage.

The Crème consisted of a fairly stiff ointment, which on analysis gave results corresponding to the following formula :

Zinc oxide	25·6 per cent.
Calcium carbonate	2·7 ,,
,, sulphate	15·8 ,,
Boric acid	15·9 ,,
Basis	58·7 ,,

The basis consisted of soft paraffin, apparently with a small proportion of a saponifiable oil, such as olive oil.

The estimated cost of the ingredients for 4 ounces is 1½d.

Paciderma Powder.—Price 9d. per box, containing about 3 ounces. The directions ran :

Allays all itching and irritation, and should be applied freely and frequently to the affected parts, in fact whenever they itch or irritate.

Analysis showed the composition to be :

Maize starch	54 per cent.
Boric acid	14 ,,
Insoluble mineral matter	19 ,,
Moisture	13 ,,

The insoluble mineral matter contained alumina, magnesia, and silica, corresponding to a mixture of talc and kaolin; this composition also agreed with all its other properties.

The estimated cost of ingredients for 3 ounces is ¾d.

Paciderma Blood Wafers.—Price 2s. 9d. per box of thirty.

Directions. One to be taken every night at bedtime.

The "wafers" consisted of cachets, each containing about 8¼ grains of a powder, the composition of which was indicated by analysis to be :

Sodium bicarbonate	59 per cent.
Precipitated sulphur	37 ,,
Powdered ginger	3 ,,
Aloin	1 ,,

The ginger and aloin could only be estimated approximately.

The estimated cost of the ingredients for 30 wafers is one-fifth of a penny.

CUTICURA REMEDIES.

The remedies are stated to be prepared by a Drug and Chemical Corporation in the U.S.A.

The "system," which has been very widely advertised, consists of Cuticura (Ointment), Cuticura Soap, and Cuticura Resolvent (liquid or pills); the ointment and the resolvent liquid were taken for analysis.

A booklet was enclosed in each package, containing, with other matter, directions for the use of the remedies in fourteen languages; from it the following extracts are taken:

In the treatment of torturing, disfiguring, itching, scaly, crusted, pimply, blotchy, and scrofulous humours of the skin, scalp, and blood, with loss of hair the Cuticura Remedies have been wonderfully successful. Even the most obstinate of constitutional humours, such as bad blood, scrofula, inherited and contagious humours, with loss of hair, glandular swellings, ulcerous patches in the throat and mouth, sore eyes, copper-coloured blotches, as well as boils, carbuncles, sties, ulcers, scrofulous rheumatism, and most humours arising from an impure or impoverished condition of the blood, yield to the CUTICURA SYSTEM OF TREATMENT in the majority of cases, when the usual remedies fail. . . . Parents are assured that these Remedies are composed of the purest and sweetest ingredients known to modern pharmacy, and may be used on the youngest infants with complete satisfaction.

Cuticura Ointment.—Price 2s. 6d. per box, containing 1¾ ounces.

Directions. . . . Cuticura Ointment may be applied to any part of the surface of the body by direct application with the finger, the palm of the hand, or spread on cotton, linen, or absorbent cotton, and covered with a light bandage, or by any means by which a remedy of this consistence would be used.

. . . in rare instances of individual tendency to acute eczema, acne, acne rosacea, erysipelas, and other highly inflammatory conditions, especially those affecting the face, it may act as an irritant, and hence those using it must observe what has been said in the foregoing directions in order that they may exercise judgment as to whether to continue it or not, should any unfavourable symptom present itself.

Examination of the ointment showed the absence of all metallic compounds, also of alkaloids or other active principles, and of saponifiable fat. It consisted of a mixture of hard and soft paraffins, slightly perfumed with rose, and coloured green. The chief green colouring matter present appeared to be an aniline dye, and a mixture of paraffins, coloured with a trace of malachite green and a little chlorophyll, agreed very closely with it in its properties. No other ingredient could be discovered.

The estimated cost of the ingredients of 1¾ ounces is ¾d.

Cuticura Resolvent.—Price 2s. 6d. per bottle, containing 6½ fluid ounces.

In the pamphlet quoted above it is stated:

> Cuticura Resolvent is alterative, antiseptic, tonic, digestive, and aperient, and is confidently believed to be superior to other preparations for purifying the system of humours of the skin, scalp, and blood, with loss of hair. CUTICURA RESOLVENT is prepared in accordance with the most advanced pharmaceutical and therapeutical knowledge from medicinal agents of ascertained purity and potency, and while in the highest degree effective, commends itself to delicate, sensitive, and refined people, especially women, because of its pure, sweet, and gentle action. . . . It is believed to be one of the most successful of blood-purifying and strengthening medicines for children in all conditions which point to inherited impurities and weaknesses, and may be taken on the first appearance of glandular swellings, ulcers, sores, especially on the neck, pallor, weakness, and delicate, frail conditions, with every hope of success.
>
> DIRECTIONS.—Adult dose, two teaspoonfuls three times a day; for children over ten years of age and delicate females, one teaspoonful; for children from five to ten years of age, one half of a teaspoonful; for children two to five years of age, 15 drops; from one to two years, 10 drops. To be taken three times a day, immediately after each meal.

Analysis showed the composition of the mixture to be:

Potassium iodide	17 grains.
Sugar and glucose	486 „
Extractive	8 „
Alcohol	10 fluid drachms.
Water to	6½ fluid ounces.

No alkaloidal substance was present; the extractive gave a slight indication of the presence of a preparation of rhubarb; all other drugs with well-marked characters were absent.

ZAM-BUK.

This ointment is sold by a London Company in a box, containing three-fifths of an ounce, price 1s. 1½d.; a Zam-Buk soap is also recommended for use as part of the treatment. In a circular enclosed in the package it was related how:

> Certain medicinal plants were taken, and from them were extracted gums and juices possessing considerable healing and curative power. Costly

experiments at last secured the right blending of these juices; and to the final product, a preparation virtually capable of growing new and healthy skin, the name of Zam-Buk was given. . . . .

Zam-Buk practically contains those substances which Nature has intended for the use of man ever since she bequeathed to him the instinct to rub a place that hurts. . . .

Zam-Buk has proved itself to be unequalled for Cuts, Bruises, Burns, Scalds Abrasions, Festering Sores, Poisoned Wounds, Lacerated Wounds, Old Wounds, Sprains, Strains, Swellings, Dog Bites, Cat Scratches, Obstinate Sores, Chafings, Itch (Scabies), Stings from Hornets, Bees, Wasps, Centipedes, and Spiders; Running Sores, Ulcers, Ringworm, Eczema (acute or chronic form), Psoriasis (tetter), Pimples, Acne, Abscesses, Boils, Carbuncles, Scrofula, Cramp, Barber's Itch, Heat Rashes, Sunburn, Freckles, Blotches, Blackheads, Scalp Irritations, Scurf or Dandruff, and other Scalp Sores; Colds, Chills, Raw Chapped Hands, Sore Lips, Raw Chin after Shaving; Inflamed Patches, Sore Nipples, Glandular Swellings, Swollen Knees, Bad Legs, Blind and Bleeding Piles, Cold-Sores, Sore Backs, Diseased or Weak Ankles, Sore and Aching Feet, Perspiring Feet, Chilblains, Soft Corns, Saltwater Sores. Rubbed well into the part affected, Zam-Buk gives great relief from Rheumatism, Lumbago, Neuralgia, Sciatica, Toothache, and allays all kinds of Inflammation, Itching, and Irritation.

The directions on the box were:

For Bruises, Cuts, Sores, Sprains, Open Wounds, Sore Breasts, Inflamed Patches, Ulcers, Eczema and Piles; first cleanse the parts with pure water and then apply Zam-Buk direct or on a piece of clean lint. For Burns, Scalds, etc., rub Zam-Buk lightly over the injured part and cover same as soon as possible in order to exclude the air. To use Zam-Buk as an Embrocation rub it in well, both into the muscles and tendons, when the healing, stimulating and strengthening ingredients in Zam-Buk will be absorbed into the system.

Analysis showed its composition to be:

Oil of eucalyptus	14 per cent. (approximately)
Pale resin (colophony)	20 ,, ,,
Soft paraffin	55 ,, ,,
Hard paraffin	11 ,, ,,
Green colouring matter	a trace.

An ointment prepared in accordance with this formula and tinted with chlorophyll agreed in all respects with the original.

The estimated cost of the ingredients for three-fifths of an ounce is ¼d.

ZIP OINTMENT.

This is supplied by a Company giving an address in a London suburb in box containing rather less than an ounce (0·85 ounce), at the price of 1s. 1½d.

On a circular enclosed with the box this ointment was described as a "cure for Eczema, Ringworm, Psoriasis." It was also stated that:

Zip is the product of many years' experience and trials, and will be found the best and most reliable remedy for the above troublesome complaints.

The directions given on the box were:

Wash well the parts with the Zip Skin Soap, and apply Zip night and morning.

Analysis showed the composition of the ointment to be:

Calomel	2·1 parts.
Lead acetate	1·0 part.
„ oleate	2·5 parts.
Oil (probably olive)	2 ,,
Glycerine	5 ,,
Creosote	A trac.
Oil of lemon grass	Sufficient to perfume.
Paraffin ointment	To 100 parts.

The estimated cost of the ingredients for 0·85 ounce is ½d.

The following are quoted from Dr. Zernik's notes on some of the skin remedies most advertised in Germany.

CRÈME EKZEMIN.

Crème Ekzemin, advertised as a cure for almost all diseases of the skin, including psoriasis, is a mixture of precipitated sulphur and a semi-fluid fatty mass, coloured red. The tube contains 75 grammes, and costs 5s. 2½d.

PHEUN SKIN PASTE.

Pheun Skin Paste, according to the vendors, possesses marvellous properties, and when applied to the skin it not only removes all the dirt but kills all the bacteria, even when situated in the deeper layers, and it is recommended as a cure for all forms of skin diseases. Zernik, on analysis, found it to contain 31 per cent. of soft paraffin, 5 per cent. of water, 2 per cent. of soap, and 10 per cent. of a dry substance yielding slimy material.

JUNIPER BEAUTY CREAM AND JUNIPER BEAUTY SOAP.

It may be worth while to add that Zernik says of a certain "Juniper Beauty Cream," sold in Berlin, that it is a water-containing ointment, perfumed with oil of bergamot, containing 5 per cent. of white precipitate (ammoniated mercury) and 11 per cent. of salicylic acid. It seems to be intended for the face, but looking to the large proportion of salicylic acid it contains, it might, perhaps, be more appropriate for use as a corn plaster.

RINO CURATIVE OINTMENT.

Rino Curative Ointment, advertised as containing naphthalan, Peru balsam, chrysarobin, etc., was found by Zernik to consist of turpentine, oil of cade, 1 per cent. of boric acid, 6 or 7 per cent. of yolk of egg and an indifferent vehicle,

CHAPTER XI.

MEDICINES FOR BALDNESS.

DURING recent years the number of preparations put forward for the cure of baldness has been increased by a new class, those, namely, which are not applied locally but taken internally. The principal ingredient in all seems to be the dried colouring matter of the blood of warm-blooded animals—haemoglobin. The most widely advertised of them is sold under the name of "Capsuloids."

CAPSULOIDS.

The price was 2s. 3d. for a box containing 36 capsuloids.

On the outer package it was stated that:

Our special process used in making Capsuloids is never used and never has been used outside our Laboratory. It is known only to the Capsuloid Company, Ltd., and has never at any time been communicated to any other person or firm. This material is then enclosed in little pear-shaped gelatine capsules which are made of the finest and purest gelatine. As a result of our special process, Capsuloids have that particular and remarkable effect upon the hair through the medium of the blood which is so well and widely known. There is no other preparation which possesses anything like the same effect.

Capsuloids not only cause the death of those harmful germs which we have proved to be the cause of falling out and prematurely grey hair, but they also restore the injured growing cells of the hair roots, and nourish them, and cause them to multiply so that the roots become firm and grow rapidly, producing thick and luxuriant hair, and where there has been premature greyness, it is also cured. Recent scientific investigation has definitely proved this, and has demonstrated that hair cannot be made to grow by using external preparations.

Directions. To stop falling out of the hair and to restore the colour to prematurely grey hair, adults should take two, or in very severe cases three, capsuloids before eating or with the first part of each meal, three times daily. The doses for younger persons is one or two with each meal. Capsuloids never cause constipation or indigestion, nor do they in any way upset the stomach, or any part of the system.

A booklet of 20 pages was enclosed in the package, in which the above statements were repeated and further elaborated with the aid of a diagram of the root of a hair, with blood-vessels, oil gland, "growing cells containing harmful germs," etc.

The capsuloids were elongated gelatine capsules containing a dark material; the average contents of one weighing 3·4 grains. The material yielded 32 per cent. to a solvent suitable for extracting fats, and this portion proved to be a mixture of about equal parts of a neutral oil and a fatty acid, agreeing in their characters with olive oil and oleic acid, respectively. Extraction of the residue with alcohol then removed 10 per cent. of an aromatic balsamic substance, generally resembling Peruvian balsam, but lighter in colour; a mixture of equal parts of Peruvian balsam and purified storax gave a substance practically identical. The residue, insoluble in both solvents, was a red-brown powder, which was found by its characters to be dried haemoglobin. Careful search was made for arsenic, alkaloids, and other ingredients, but nothing else was detected. The results indicated the following formula for the contents of the capsules :

Haemoglobin	1·97 grain.
Olive oil ⎱ of each .... Oleic acid ⎰	0 54 ,,
Balsam of Peru ⎱ of each .... Purified storax ⎰	0·17 ,,
In one capsule.	

The estimated cost of materials for the contents of 36 capsules is 1d.

Other dealers have paid the company the sincere compliment of imitation, and various similar articles appear to be largely sold. The following particulars are taken from price lists and advertisements intended for retail chemists; as haemoglobin is referred to as the principal constituent in each case, they were not submitted to analysis.

CAPSULATED HAEMOGLOBIN OVALS FOR THE HAIR.

"Capsulated Haemoglobin Ovals for the Hair. Contain 2½ grains of Pure Haemoglobin."

They were supplied by a firm in a south country seaside town, labelled with name and address of the retailer. The wholesale price quoted was for tubes of 25, 4s. per dozen.

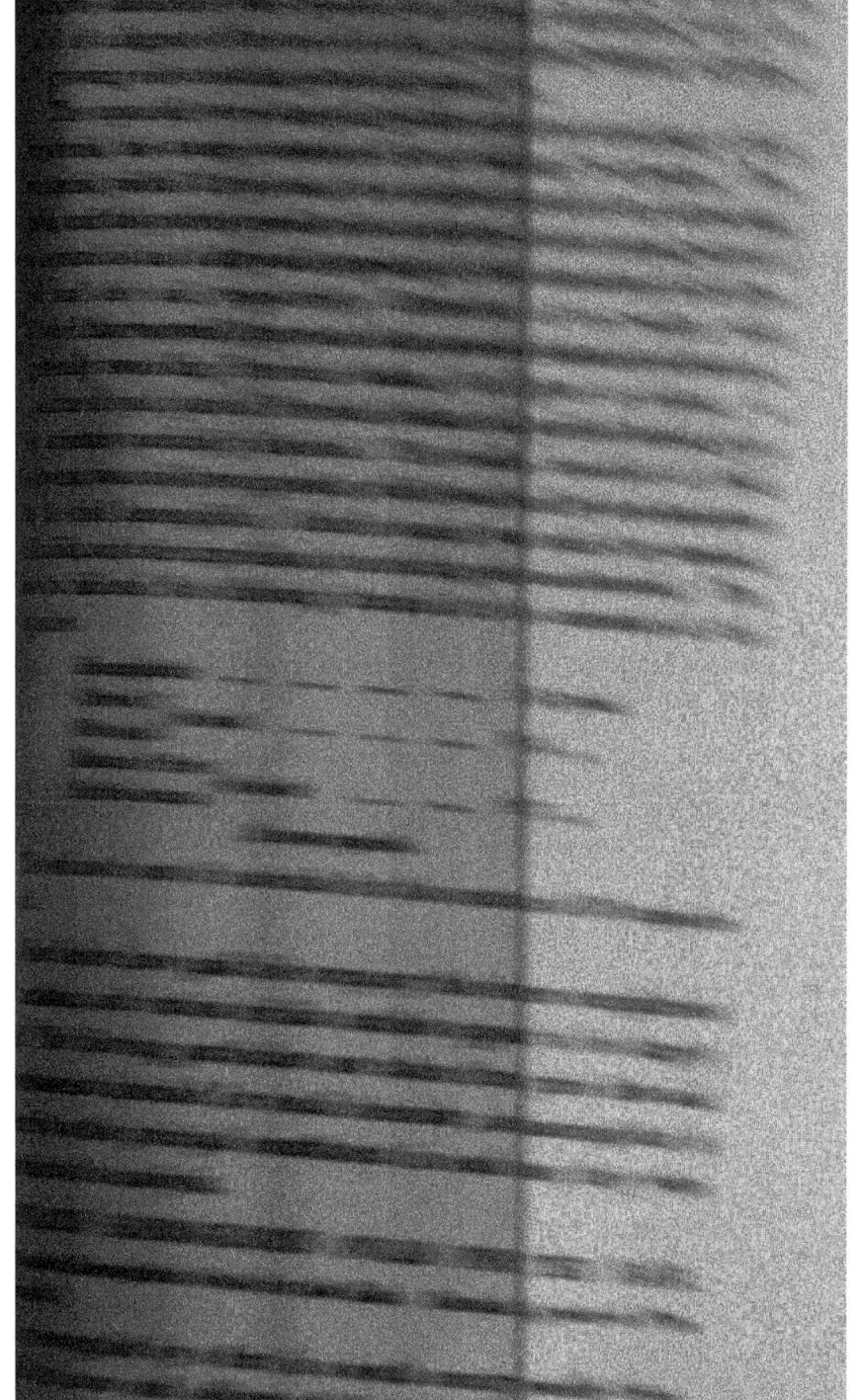

CHAPTER XI.

MEDICINES FOR BALDNESS.

DURING recent years the number of preparations put forward for the cure of baldness has been increased by a new class, those, namely, which are not applied locally but taken internally. The principal ingredient in all seems to be the dried colouring matter of the blood of warm-blooded animals—haemoglobin. The most widely advertised of them is sold under the name of "Capsuloids."

CAPSULOIDS.

The price was 2s. 3d. for a box containing 36 capsuloids.

On the outer package it was stated that:

Our special process used in making Capsuloids is never used and never has been used outside our Laboratory. It is known only to the Capsuloid Company, Ltd., and has never at any time been communicated to any other person or firm. This material is then enclosed in little pear-shaped gelatine capsules which are made of the finest and purest gelatine. As a result of our special process, Capsuloids have that particular and remarkable effect upon the hair through the medium of the blood which is so well and widely known. There is no other preparation which possesses anything like the same effect.

Capsuloids not only cause the death of those harmful germs which we have proved to be the cause of falling out and prematurely grey hair, but they also restore the injured growing cells of the hair roots, and nourish them, and cause them to multiply so that the roots become firm and grow rapidly, producing thick and luxuriant hair, and where there has been premature greyness, it is also cured. Recent scientific investigation has definitely proved this, and has demonstrated that hair cannot be made to grow by using external preparations.

Directions. To stop falling out of the hair and to restore the colour to prematurely grey hair, adults should take two, or in very severe cases three, capsuloids before eating or with the first part of each meal, three times daily. The doses for younger persons is one or two with each meal. Capsuloids never cause constipation or indigestion, nor do they in any way upset the stomach, or any part of the system.

A booklet of 20 pages was enclosed in the package, in which the above statements were repeated and further elaborated with the aid of a diagram of the root of a hair, with blood-vessels, oil gland, " growing cells containing harmful germs," etc.

The capsuloids were elongated gelatine capsules containing a dark material, the average contents of one weighing 3·4 grains. The material yielded 32 per cent. to a solvent suitable for extracting fats, and this portion proved to be a mixture of about equal parts of a neutral oil and a fatty acid, agreeing in their characters with olive oil and oleic acid, respectively. Extraction of the residue with alcohol then removed 10 per cent. of an aromatic balsamic substance, generally resembling Peruvian balsam, but lighter in colour; a mixture of equal parts of Peruvian balsam and purified storax gave a substance practically identical. The residue, insoluble in both solvents, was a red-brown powder, which was found by its characters to be dried haemoglobin. Careful search was made for arsenic, alkaloids, and other ingredients, but nothing else was detected. The results indicated the following formula for the contents of the capsules :

Haemoglobin	1·97 grain.
Olive oil ⎱ of each .... Oleic acid ⎰	0 54 ,,
Balsam of Peru ⎱ of each .... Purified storax ⎰	0·17 ,,
In one capsule.	

The estimated cost of materials for the contents of 36 capsules is 1d.

Other dealers have paid the company the sincere compliment of imitation, and various similar articles appear to be largely sold. The following particulars are taken from price lists and advertisements intended for retail chemists ; as haemoglobin is referred to as the principal constituent in each case, they were not submitted to analysis.

CAPSULATED HAEMOGLOBIN OVALS FOR THE HAIR.

" Capsulated Haemoglobin Ovals for the Hair. Contain 2¼ grains of Pure Haemoglobin."

They were supplied by a firm in a south country seaside town, labelled with name and address of the retailer. The wholesale price quoted was for tubes of 25, 4s. per dozen.

HAEMOGLOBIN HAIR CAPSULES.

"Capsules for the Hair. When falling out or turning prematurely grey, these capsules by enriching the blood make the hair glossy, luxuriant, and full of vitality."

These were not described on the package as containing haemoglobin, but were quoted in the price list as "Haemoglobin Hair Capsules." They were supplied by a company in a seaside town. "Store price, 1s. 6d." Wholesale price, 7s. per dozen packages.

SOLUBLE CAPSULES OF HAEMOGLOBIN.

"Soluble Capsules of Haemoglobin. A natural hair food. Produces Healthy, Strong, and Luxuriant Hair."

The wholesale price of these, supplied by a London firm, was for boxes of 36, 5s. 9d. per dozen.

CHAPTER XII.

CANCER REMEDIES.

A VERY slight acquaintance with the advertisements of quack medicines is enough to show that a knowledge of the causes of the disease for which a cure is promised is in no wise necessary for the composition of either the medicine or the advertisement; in fact, it is impossible to believe that the extravagant claims and absurd statements made could be put forward by persons having any knowledge of disease. It is no matter for surprise, therefore, that in the case of the least understood and least successfully combated of diseases many proprietary " remedies " are put forward. A considerable number of these articles have been received and the alleged claims tested at the laboratories of the Imperial Cancer Research Fund; specimens of a few of these were obtained and submitted to analysis, and some notes on their composition cannot fail to be of interest to members of the medical profession, who will probably from time to time have to treat sufferers from cancer who have been induced to buy one or other of these preparations.

As was to be expected, the articles examined have little or nothing in common. In the case of diseases for which the ordinary treatment involves the use of certain specific drugs, proprietary medicines are usually merely varying compounds of those drugs; thus, of the advertised cures for epilepsy, analyses of which are given in the next chapter, the essential ingredient in all but one is an alkaline bromide. But in cancer the would-be maker of a proprietary " cure " has no such accepted treatment to guide him, or to restrict the free range of his fancy in selection of ingredients; it is probable that some of the " remedies " here described were inspired by the fact that some apparent improvement followed their fortuitous use in some cases, *post hoc* having been assumed to mean *propter hoc;* the first to be described, however, can hardly rest even on this basis.

It is a colourless liquid, containing a trace of sediment; the odour is that of alcohol, though very slightly vinous. Fractional distillation showed the presence of about 40 per cent. of alcohol; on complete evaporation, a trace (0·02 per cent.) of dry residue was left. This residue was free from any alkaloid, and its behaviour with reagents gave no indication of any other active principle; it agreed in character with the "extractive" found in spirit that has been kept in a wine-cask. After removing the alcohol, the liquid was perfectly tasteless. This "remedy" is thus very simple in nature, consisting merely of diluted and slightly impure alcohol. Its composition brings to mind the analysis published some years ago of a so-called electric fluid, or "electricity," for the cure of cancer, which was taken up by a certain well-known journalist and boomed by him in the pages of the review which he edited; many marvellous cures were ascribed to it, but examination showed that although it was sold at several shillings per fluid ounce, it consisted of plain water. Notwithstanding the exposure, the article is at present quoted in wholesale lists, and is therefore presumably still in demand. The cost of the "medicine" we are now dealing with is of course considerably greater than the cost of plain water, but this fact will be but small consolation to the victim who derives as little benefit from the one as from the other.

The next article analysed was a blue fluid containing a considerable blue sediment, and smelling fairly strongly of terebene. The chief ingredient was found to be a blue dye stuff of the oxazine or thiazine group, much resembling methylene blue (which is the only member of these groups ordinarily used in medicine), but differing from it in solubility and in its behaviour with certain reagents. This constituted the greater part of the sediment, and a portion of the dye was also in solution. The liquid further contained a dissolved gum and a trace of terebene; these, with a little magnesium carbonate, were all the ingredients present. No trace of any alkaloid was found, and the solvent was water. The gum showed no difference from ordinary acacia gum, and was probably added to suspend the undissolved dye stuff. Water dissolves very little terebene, and no more of the latter was present than could be dissolved by the water; it was probably employed to give an aromatic taste and smell, and the magnesia was doubtless used to subdivide the terebene in the manner commonly followed by pharmacists when dissolving essential oils in water. It thus appears that the essential ingredient of this medicine is the blue dye stuff; it is possible that this has been used as methylene blue, since the articles sent out under the same name by different dye manufacturers often differ in composition; but, as already stated, it is not identical with the methylene blue usually met with. The total solids in the mixture, after shaking up the sediment, amounted to 13·2 per cent., of which the dye stuff constituted something like one-half.

A third preparation was a brown liquid of syrupy consistence found to consist of wood tar. It was a much purer product than ordinary Stockholm tar, and its peculiar odour indicated that it was derived, at least in great part, from the birch; no other ingredient could be found. This article came from Sphakia, Crete; the label bore no directions for its use, leaving it uncertain whether it was intended for internal or external use, but the latter appears the more probable.

The remaining articles are clearly intended for external application; the first of these consisted of a plaster mass, in the half-pound sticks in which such masses are usually supplied. Analysis showed the principal ingredient to be lead oleate, with a little stearate, and small quantities of resin and soap. These are the ingredients of the resin and the soap plasters of the *British Pharmacopœia*, and the proportion of soap present showed the specimen under examination to be emplastrum resinae.

The next preparation was an ointment of Dutch origin. It contained large quantities of ammonium alum and zinc sulphate, with a little sodium sulphate, made up into a stiff ointment with a basis consisting of beeswax, soft paraffin, oil, and resin. The quantities of the salts were approximately:

Alum	27 per cent.
Zinc sulphate	37 ,,
Sodium sulphate	8 ,,

The presence of so large a proportion of mineral salts, of course, leaves very little tenacity in the ointment; particles of the white salts were easily visible to the eye, and the effect of applying the preparation must be practically the same as if the dry salts were rubbed on the skin except that the basis would, of course, act as a lubricant in the rubbing.

The last of these preparations was another ointment; the mineral ingredients in this case, however, were in organic combination. This ointment contained copper oleate and aluminium oleate with a basis of lard and a little resin. The proportions of the active ingredients were approximately:

Copper oleate	15 per cent.
Aluminium oleate	35 ,,

No alkaloid or other active principle was found.

A bottle of lotion for cancer and other affections, obtained in the ordinary way through a dealer, was examined. The label commences with the statement that the lotion " cures cancerous or malignant sores "; then follows a list of other diseases, with the addition, " even cases that have been under the treatment of doctors and at infirmaries for years." Analysis showed the composition of the lotion to be substantially as follows:—

Zinc sulphate	92 grains.
Carbolic acid (pure phenol)	1·2 oz.
Glycerine	1·8 fl. oz.
Cochineal solution sufficient to give a deep red colour.	
Water to 3·3 fl. oz.	

This quantity is contained in a bottle costing 4s. 6d.; the directions are to add the whole contents to 1½ pints of water, which is to be applied to the diseased parts for about five minutes two or three times a day.

Another pretended "cure" for this disease was supplied from an address in Croydon, by a person who described himself as a retired Government analytical chemist. The bottle did not bear an Inland Revenue stamp. The vendor seems to prefer to see and examine the patients. In one such case he was paid 3 guineas, and asked for more, as it was, he said, a complicated case. The directions given were "two tablespoonfuls should be taken three times a day." Analysis of this liquid showed the presence of ferric chloride, and traces of hydrochloric acid and alcohol, and nothing else except water; the alcohol indicates that the tincture of perchloride of iron, and not the liquor, was employed; determination of the amounts of iron and chlorine present showed that 6 fluid ounces of the mixture contained 5·7 fluid drachms of the tincture.

A few years ago a good deal was heard of the wonderful cures said to be achieved by two persons who resided at Cardigan. A great deal of secrecy was observed, but it was known that a fluid was applied to the surface of the cancerous tumour. The treatment, it was stated, began with prayer, and exhortations to the patient to trust in the Almighty; the lotion or oil, which was said to be made entirely from herbs and to contain no mineral caustic, was then painted on with a brush. Unlike other empirics who profess to remove the "roots" which the knife leaves behind, these Welsh practitioners asserted that their remedy made the "roots" shrink into the original growth which then fell off like a ripe apple from a tree. The practice seemed to be to require the patient to attend daily to have the local applications made for periods extending over several months. Eventually, in some cases, a mass of dried, heaped-up crusts formed, and when this became detached it was put into a bottle and given to the patient who was told that it was the cancer extracted by the treatment. In one case which was enquired into, this bottled cancer was submitted to microscopical examination; it was found to consist of crusts formed of sloughing parts of the skin and inflammatory exudation, the whole being such a mass as might be produced by the use of an escharotic. The crusts when submitted to chemical analysis were found to contain zinc chloride in considerable amount, together with a very appreciable quantity of an insoluble compound of lead. A healing oil was also supplied to help the cancer falling off, and this when chemically examined was found to contain 27 per cent. of oil of turpentine, the remainder consisting principally of an ordinary saponifiable oil, probably cotton-seed or olive oil. In addition there was a considerable amount of deposit which proved to consist almost wholly of barium sulphate, a very insoluble salt, used, under the name of permanent white, by water-colour artists. It would seem, therefore, that the statement that the applications contained no mineral caustic was inaccurate. In other patients the effect of this Cardigan treatment was more destructive. In the case of one woman who had been informed that the cancer had been cured and that she only required some tonic medicine to complete the cure, the surgeon who was called to her when she was *in extremis* has said that he never beheld anything like it in his life; the whole breast was a necrosing mass, black and stinking, the ulcers extending up to the collar-bone and down to the margin of the ribs and across the middle line; the hand could have been inserted under the margin of the dead part all round. Some unfortunate patients persevered with the treatment although suffering pain described as excruciating.

Caustics are, in fact, the weapon of the quack, and although they may have a legitimate sphere in surgery, it is very limited; zinc chloride, for instance, has occasionally been used in a strong solution or paste as a caustic under special circumstances. Although portions of a tumour may be removed by caustic application, it is impossible to eradicate the whole in this way, as the cancerous process is extending into adjacent parts. The formula of the quack—" cancer treated without the knife "—appeals with great force to the public who do not know the terrible long-drawn-out agony which those treated with caustics have to undergo. Of this a vivid description was given by a well-known naturalist, the father of a distinguished man of letters, in a little book in which he related the suffering of his own wife; she was treated by an American cancer-curer by caustics. The process of " cure" lasted several months, and the result may be summed up in the statement that "suffering never ceased from the beginning of the operation till her spirit was freed from the worn-out body."

CHAPTER XIII.

REMEDIES FOR EPILEPSY.

THE nostrums which appear to be most advertised at the present time for the treatment of epilepsy afford a good example of the fact which has been previously pointed out that in some instances the vendors of secret preparations make use of drugs in common use by the medical profession for the treatment of some particular disorder; this is, of course, only possible when the symptoms are well-marked and easily recognised. As will be seen from the analyses given below of a number of nostrums advertised as remedies for epilepsy it was found that all, with one exception, contained bromide salts, that is to say, a drug the effect of which is described and discussed in every medical work dealing with the disease; nevertheless, the advertisers endeavour to lead the purchaser to believe that the preparations possess peculiar virtues unknown to the medical profession. The exceptional preparation contains vervain (*Verbena officinalis*) which held a place in the old pharmacopœias and herbals, chiefly as an astringent application to wounds or as a lotion for sore mouth. Dodoens (1572) says it is good for headache applied as a plaster, while Gerarde (1633) mentions its use as a garland round the head for the same condition, but he disapproves of the many old wives' tales told regarding it which tend to sorcery, and are such as honest ears abhor to hear; indeed, he hints that some assert that the "divell did reveal it as a secret and divine medicine." According to Pliny, vervain was gathered by the Druids of Gaul and Britain at the rising of the Dog Star, when neither sun nor moon shone, with the left hand only, and after libations of honey. When thus obtained it was said to vanquish fevers and other distempers, to be an antidote to the bite of serpents, and a charm to conciliate friendship. Paris speaks of it as in his own time the subject of a work on scrofula by a Mr. Morley, which was written for the sole purpose of restoring the much injured character and use of vervain, so that it is evidently a herb which has suffered much from detraction. Mr. Morley directed the root of the plant to be tied, with a yard of white satin ribbon, round the neck where it was to remain until the patient was cured. The modern vendor does not indulge in these refinements.

In submitting the following analyses it should be stated that a mixture or powder, dispensed according to the prescription obtained by the analysis, produced in each case a preparation closely resembling in appearance and taste that sold by the secret medicine vendor; further, the mixtures possessed the same specific gravity as the originals.

OZERINE.

"Ozerine," prepared by a chemist in Ireland, is described as an unfailing remedy for epilepsy, fits, or falling sickness. The bottle examined had no medicine stamp affixed.

The formula ascertained by analysis is as follows:

Potassium bromide	120 grains.
Ammonium carbonate	16 ,,
Burnt sugar	q.s. to colour.
Chloroform water to 1 fluid ounce.	

Potassium bromide (111 grains) and potassium chloride ($9\frac{1}{3}$ grains) were found by analysis, but as some potassium bromide containing a large percentage of chloride had recently been in the market the latter was not regarded as an intentional addition.

Dose.—One teaspoonful before breakfast and dinner, and two at bedtime.

The price charged for a bottle containing 8 fluid ounces was 4s. 6d.; the estimated cost of contents was under 4d.

W. AND J. TAYLOR'S CELEBRATED ANTI-EPILEPTIC MEDICINE.

This preparation, sold in this country through an export agent in London, is said to be "simple, efficacious, harmless, and cheap." The effrontery of the following paragraph, extracted from a circular which was wrapped round the bottle, is amusing in view of the analytical results:

> The principal drug is to be found in nearly every surgery, and yet not one doctor in a hundred would think of using it in Epilepsy, simply because he has no precedent to act upon—he is not directed by any of the great medical writers to prescribe or administer it in this disease; he knows not of its being so used, and he has not tried it himself, and thus he remains unaware of the one grand means of curing Epilepsy, even with the very drugs necessary at his elbow.

The formula ascertained by analysis was:

Tincture of iodine	$\frac{3}{4}$ minim.
Potassium bromide	13 grains.
Ammonium bromide	4 ,,
Water to 1 fluid ounce.	

The mixture contained the proportion of iodine indicated in the above formula; but as it also contained traces of iodide, it was probable that tincture of iodine was used in its preparation. It may, however, have been prepared from an aqueous solution of iodine and potassium iodide.

Dose.—One teaspoonful three times a day.

The price of a bottle holding 12 fluid ounces was 2s. 9d.; the estimated cost of the contents is about 1d.

OSBORNE'S MIXTURE FOR EPILEPSY.

This mixture is stated to be prepared in a small town in England.

The following is an extract from a circular accompanying the bottle:

> It scarcely ever fails to prevent the fits, loss of consciousness, convulsions, nervous twitchings, &c., of epilepsy, while at the same time it acts as a most valuable tonic; it allays irritation of the nervous system, purifies the blood, strengthens the frame, improves the general health, and helps to check the progress of disease on the intellectual faculties, and may be taken by the most delicate.

The formula ascertained by analysis was:

Potassium bromide	....	166 grains.
Sugar	....	48 ,, (= syrup ʒj).
Burnt sugar	....	q.s. to colour.
Peppermint water to 1 fluid ounce.		

Traces of fixed ammonia were also present.

Dose.—One large teaspoonful morning and night.

The price charged for a bottle holding 5 fluid ounces was 2s. 9d.; the estimated cost of the contents is about 3d.

"PROFESSOR" O. PHELPS BROWN'S VERVAIN RESTORATIVE ASSIMILANT.

This preparation is recommended by the vendor—

"for the positive and speedy cure of epilepsy or fits, dyspepsia, indigestion, all derangements of the stomach and bowels, and for every form of debility, no matter from what source it may arise. An unequalled tonic and nervine."

The formula ascertained by analysis was:

Decoction of Vervain (2 oz. to a pint)	4 fluid drachms.
Port wine	1 ,, ,,
Rectified spirit	2 ,, ,,
Water to 1 fluid ounce.	

The dose was stated to be one dessertspoonful three times a day before eating.

The mixture contained 25·75 per cent. of absolute alcohol by volume, and reacted towards lead acetate and lead subacetate exactly like a specimen prepared according to the above formula. It also contained the same amount of extractive, and had the same specific gravity.

The price is 2s. 9d. for a 6-oz. bottle. The estimated cost of the contents is about 5d.

TRENCH'S REMEDY FOR EPILEPSY AND FITS.

This is, or was, made by a company giving an address in Ireland. The package examined had no medicine stamp affixed.

Liquid Preparation.—The following formula refers to the liquid preparation supplied for use in the United Kingdom.

The formula ascertained by analysis was:

Potassium bromide	....	....	....	70 grains.		
Ammonium bromide	....	....	....	10 ,,		
Sugar	....	....	....	....	....	72 ,, (= syrup ʒjss).
Fuchsin q.s. to colour.						
Water to 1 fluid ounce.						

The dose was stated to be one teaspoonful in the morning and two at night; the price for a 3-oz. bottle is 3s.; the estimated cost of the contents was about 1d.

"*Concentrated Form.*"—This was supplied for export to the colonies, was a moist coarse brown crystalline powder in hermetically-sealed tins, with directions enclosed for dissolving in water. A quarter package (the smallest supplied) contained 11¼ ounces, and was directed to be dissolved in one pint of warm water. The resulting mixture was found to measure 25 fluid ounces. From the formula given below it will be seen that the mixture thus prepared differed from the one issued for home consumption in two important particulars: (*a*) ammonium bromide was absent, (*b*) the dose of potassium bromide was considerably larger than that of the total bromides in the latter. Is this a form of colonial preference? or is it that our brothers beyond the sea are more robust and hence proof against the depressing influence of potassium salts? The formula of the powder ascertained by analysis was:

Potassium bromide	....	....	....	61 parts.
Moist brown sugar	....	....	....	39 ,,

The calculated composition of the finished mixture was:

Potassium bromide	....	....	....	120 grains.
Moist brown sugar	....	....	....	77 ,,
Water to 1 fluid ounce.				

The dose of the mixture directed to be taken was one teaspoonful in the morning and two at night.

The price charged for a quarter package was 15s., but the estimated cost of the contents is about 8d.

Such then are these secret remedies for epilepsy; with one exception they are weak preparations of well known drugs supplied at considerably more than the usual cost, and administered without that careful adjustment of dose to the needs of the particular patient which is, after all, the most essential part in the treatment of epilepsy by bromide salts. The exception contains an old-fashioned herb once praised by the superstitious but abandoned time and again even by them; it has never been shown to possess any definite therapeutic properties and was long ago discarded by the medical profession because it was found useless.

SOME GERMAN NOSTRUMS.

Of five nostrums sold for the cure of epilepsy in Germany, examined by Dr. Zernik, three were found to contain bromide salts as chief constituents : *Lamma powder* consisted of equal parts of bromide of sodium and bromide of ammonium ; *Antiépileptique* (Uten) was a solution of potassium bromide (16 per cent.), coloured green, and containing 1 per cent. of an indifferent bitter tincture, while *Berendorf's powder for epilepsy* contained potassium bromide 53·3 per cent., borax 40·3 per cent., and zinc oxide 4 per cent., the remainder being water. Borax is a remedy occasionally used to correct some undesired effect of bromides and has sometimes been prescribed for patients who could not tolerate the bromides. Zinc oxide has, or at one time had, a certain reputation as a nerve sedative. Of the two German remedies which did not contain bromide one consisted largely of formaldehyde which is used as an antiseptic and preservative for food, and the other consisted of pills containing nothing beyond inactive powdered leaves and roots.

CHAPTER XIV.

SOOTHING, TEETHING AND COOLING POWDERS FOR INFANTS.

THE number of proprietary infants' powders that can be said to be at all widely advertised is small, but some of them are sold in very large numbers. In addition, powders for the same purpose are very largely supplied by retailers, put up by themselves; they are usually of similar composition to one or other of those here described, but there is, of course, great scope for variations in the quantity and proportion, as well as in the nature of the drugs employed. It may, perhaps, be hoped that the efforts now being made by the employment of health visitors in many towns will, by the spread of instruction as to the common-sense management of infants, gradually lead to a great diminution in the custom so prevalent among the poorer classes of dosing infants whenever the curious foods, still so commonly given, cause indigestion.

STEDMAN'S TEETHING POWDERS.

The powders "with one e" are sold from an address in the north of London in boxes, price 1s. 1½d., 2s. 9d., 4s. 6d., and 11s. The 4s. 6d. box contained 60 powders, and the 11s. box contained 216; the other sizes are stated to contain respectively 9 and 30 powders.

In a circular enclosed in the package it is stated that:

> The returns of the Registrar-General tell us that the period of Dentition is one of more than ordinary peril to the child. It is a time of most active development, a time of passing from one mode of being to another, and we may fairly congratulate ourselves when this time of Teething be passed. To

pass this time safely, and with the least risk to the child, one of "Stedman's Teething Powders" should be given about twice a week, during the whole time of Dentition, according to the directions below........

When the bowels are moved regularly and the motions of a natural yellow colour, the Powders had better be omitted for a time, unless great irritability be present, accompanied with restlessness, then a dose had better be given. Diarrhœa will generally be checked by giving a dose at the commencement of the attack.

The directions are :

When the Child is under three months of age, the Third of a Powder only is to be given; from three to six months Half a Powder may be used; when above six months a Whole Powder may be taken.

The average weight of one powder was 2·4 grains; twelve powders weighed singly had weights varying from 2·25 to 2·6 grains. Analysis showed the powder to be composed of :

Calomel	29 per cent.
Sugar of milk	71 ,, ,,

A trace of alkaloid was present also, and when extracted from the material of a large number of powders, was found to amount to only 0·016 per cent., or $\frac{1}{2500}$ grain in one powder. This trace of alkaloid did not show the behaviour of morphine, and did not give any reactions characteristic of any of the ordinary alkaloids, so far as it was possible to test for them on the minute amount available.

The estimated cost of the materials for the powders in a 4s. 6d. box is one-third of a penny.

STEEDMAN'S SOOTHING POWDERS.

The powders, "with two e's," are stated to be prepared in the south of London, and are sold in packets, price 1s. 1½d. and 2s. 9d. per packet; the 2s. 9d. packet contained twenty-four powders.

In a circular enclosed in the packet it is stated that :

The good effects of these Powders during the period of Teething have now had *Fifty Years' Experience,* during which time *Thousands of children have been relieved annually* from all those distressing symptoms which children suffer while cutting their teeth—viz., Feverish Heats, Fits, Convulsions, Sickness of Stomach and Debility, accompanied with Relaxation of the Bowels, and pale and green motions, or Inflammation of the Gums.
. . . the striking superiority both in the health and strength of those children who have taken the soothing Powders during the period of Teething has induced the Proprietor to make this MUCH-VALUED MEDICINE more generally known by this advertisement.

The directions are :

Dose.—From one to three months, the third of a Powder; from three to six months, half of a Powder; from six months and above that age, one Powder only and no more; . . .

The average weight of one powder was 2·8 grains; twelve powders weighed singly had weights varying from 1·9 to 4·5 grains. Analysis showed the powder to consist of:

Calomel	27 per cent.
Sugar	22 ,,
Maize starch	50·5 ,,
Ash....	0·5 ,,

A minute trace of alkaloid appeared to be present; the quantity was considerably less than in the Stedman's powders described above, and so small, in fact, as hardly to give positive evidence of its alkaloidal nature.

The estimated cost of the ingredients of Steedman's powders in a 2s. 9d. packet is one-eighth of a penny.

PRITCHARD'S TEETHING AND FEVER POWDERS.

The proprietors of these powders give an address in a large provincial city. The price charged is 1s. 1½d. for a box containing sixteen powders.

In a circular enclosed in the package it is stated:

The constantly increasing sale of these justly esteemed Powders proves them to be the most effectual Medicine that can be given to young children during the troublesome and anxious period of teething. By their gentle action on the Bowels, and valuable cooling properties, they allay all irritation and Feverishness, prevent Fits, Convulsions, &c., ensure refreshing and natural sleep for the child, and therefore peaceful nights for the parents.

The directions are:

From one to three months, a third of a Powder; from Three to six months, half a Powder; from six months and above that age, one Powder (not to be given if the child is relaxed).

The average weight of the powders was 2·1 grains; twelve powders weighed singly had weights varying from 1·9 to 2·3 grains. Analysis showed the powder to consist of:

Calomel	47 per cent.
Antimony oxide	0·7 ,,
Calcium phosphate	1·4 ,,
Sugar of milk	50·9 ,,

No trace of alkaloid was present.

The estimated cost of the ingredients of the powders in a 1s. 1½d. box is one-ninth of a penny.

FENNING'S CHILDREN'S COOLING POWDERS.

The proprietor gives an address in the south of England, and the prices charged are 1s. 1½d. and 2s. 9d. a box; the 2s. 9d. box contained 48 powders.

They were described in a circular enclosed with the box as :

The best medicine for infants cutting their teeth, preventing convulsions, thrush, disordered bowels, and for all the feverish diseases of infants and children.

The following directions are given :

For an Infant under *three* years of age, give *one* of Fennings' Cooling Powders mixed with a little water, or it could be thrown dry as it is into the opened mouth of the baby, and gently holding back the head for half a minute it would be swallowed.

Whenever an Infant is restless or feverishly hot from Teething, when it is griped or sick from improper food, or over-feeding; has acidity, or a disordered stomach, *one* of these Powders should be immediately given and, if necessary, repeated every day . . .

When a Child is attacked with Thrush, Measles, Hooping Cough. or Fever of any sort, always keep the feverish blood cool by giving a dose of *Fenning's Cooling Powders* every or every other day.

The powders had an average weight of 3·4 grains; twelve powders weighed singly had weights varying from 3·2 to 3·8 grains. Analysis showed the powder to consist of:

Potassium chlorate	70 per cent.
Powdered liquorice	30 ,,

The estimated cost of the ingredients of the powders in a 2s. 9d. box is one-sixth of a penny.

CHAPTER XV.

REMEDIES FOR EAR DISEASE AND DEAFNESS.

SOME of the advertisements most frequently seen headed "Deafness cured," "Eyes and Ears," "Eye Diseases cured," etc., do not refer to nostrums obtainable in the usual way through patent medicine dealers. The reader of the announcement is invited to write to the address given for particulars of special remedies, or an "interesting and convincing book post free," dealing with the cure of diseases without operation, etc. Application for particulars brings much printed matter recommending the advertiser's method, accompanied by a set of questions to be answered by the sufferer. If these answers are supplied and the fee demanded paid, medicine of some sort is sent. Medicines sold in this way, of which many other instances have been given in previous chapters, form a special class of "secret remedies," and might be said, perhaps, to come rather under the head of prescribing at a distance, but it is, to say the least, very doubtful whether the composition of the medicines supplied is modified according to the answers given to the questions, and the two kinds of quackery are not sharply separated. In the case of the preparations now to be described, one or two belong more nearly to the class just referred to than to that of ordinary " patent medicines."

We meet again the benevolent gentleman who having cured himself offers " to send particulars of remedy free," but eventually sells his treatment at a price which would seem to represent no bad profit on the outlay for materials.

We also meet the dealer who to encourage the possible buyer sends a reduced price coupon only asking in return for the names and addresses of two or three friends who suffer in like manner.

ALFRED CROMPTON'S SPECIFIC FOR DEAFNESS.

This so-called specific, prepared in a town in the north of England, is sold in a bottle containing half a fluid ounce, and costing 1s. 1½d. The label on the outside of the package was headed:

Deafness Cured!

and continues:

Alfred Crompton's Specific for Deafness, Noises in the Ears, &c., is decidedly the best remedy out for this most annoying complaint. A single Bottle has in most instances effected a speedy and permanent cure.

The directions were:

Warm the Specific and Shake the Bottle. Two or three drops to be dropped in the Ear, night and morning, and rub behind and under the Ear with the Specific.

Analysis showed the following composition:

Soap	3·6 per cent.
Glycerine	45·0 ,,
Oil	21·7 ,,
Water	29·5 ,,
Alcohol	a trace.
Oil of rosemary	,,

There was a slight indication of a trace of camphor; probably this with the alcohol and oil of rosemary and part of the soap were added in the form of soap liniment. The oil gave analytical figures corresponding to a mixture of almond and colza oils in about equal proportions.

The estimated cost of ingredients, for ½-oz., is one farthing.

DELLAR'S ESSENCE FOR DEAFNESS.

This so-called essence, prepared it is stated by a company giving an address in London, and sold at the price of 1s. 1½d. for a bottle, containing two-fifths of a fluid ounce, is described on the label as "An old-established and valuable remedy."

Directions for Use.—A small piece of wool, well moistened with the Essence, to be pushed into the cavity of the Ear every night at bedtime, and removed in the morning.

Analysis showed the composition to be:

Oil of turpentine	16 per cent.
Fixed oil	84 ,,

The properties of the fixed oil and the figures which it gave on further analysis corresponded to those of almond oil.

The estimated cost of the ingredients, for two-fifths of an ounce, is one halfpenny.

HERBERT CLIFTON'S TREATMENT FOR DEAFNESS.

This is brought to the notice of the public by an advertisement in the following terms:

A new cure for deafness. A Gentleman who cured himself after 14 years' suffering will send particulars of remedy free.

Here followed the gentleman's address, and an application brought a letter and a pamphlet entitled "Deafness and Noises in the Head, with Instructions how they may be Absolutely Cured," which was marked "40th edition." It professed to give an account of the writer's own experiences. A few extracts will suffice to give an idea of it:

Those only who have suffered from the terrible calamity of deafness can understand the misery it brings into one's life; and only those who have had occasion to seek the assistance of men who profess to cure this awful affliction can appreciate how utterly its treatment is misunderstood by the various advertising empirics who profess to cure it, whether by electrical, galvanic, or any of the other methods which are so alluringly set forth as perfectly infallible by people who never suffered themselves, who can have no sympathy, therefore, with those whom they profess to assist, and whose only object is to extract as large a sum as they possibly can from the pockets of those whom they have been able to attract to their spider's parlour. The writer, however, of the present pamphlet is in a different position. . . As a lad I began to suffer from noises in the head, which as time went on increased to such an alarming degree that I was taken to an Aural Surgeon. . . . The usual result followed. I became worse and worse, and, of course, weaker through his treatment. . . . Another doctor was consulted. . . . But the treatment failed, my affliction increased, and MY LIFE BECAME A BURDEN. . . . There seemed no hope for me. Nearly a dozen eminent surgeons had seen me, examined me, said different things about me, and indifferently treated me; but all to no purpose. . . . As a last resource I tried the various quack remedies which have allured so many to their bitter cost, and many a pound was wasted on mechanical, electrical, magnetic, and other useless appliances, and upon ear-trumpets, drums, tubes, &c., with no result. . . . Then the wild, yet happy, thought flashed across me: "Why not try and cure yourself?" I pondered and pondered over the idea, and at last, rather than submit to my fate, determined to study physiology and medicine and endeavour to discover the cause of my deafness, with the distant hope that I might alight upon the method of its cure. . . . The conclusion I came to was that what I really required was a medicine which should reach the minute muscles of the inner ear, as upon their proper action the sense of hearing almost entirely depends. . . . after a time I had succeeded in discovering a preparation which would do the required work. . . . My disease was of so long standing, that I had found it had caused the drums of my ears to become weak and shrunken . . . and I soon devised a small appliance to fit inside each ear—the appliance which I now term the "Invisible Drum Support" . . . in my gratitude to the Almighty for my merciful deliverance I vowed that I would publish to the world the method by which I had struggled out of the dark past into the brilliant light of the present.

A postscript to the letter stated that "No charge whatever is made for advice, so you need not hesitate to avail yourself of the benefit of my *opinion*," but no information was vouchsafed as to the price charged for the "treatment," except that it would be found extremely moderate. Paragraphs, of the usual inspired kind, were quoted from the *Family Doctor, Christian Union, Family Churchman, Health*, and local newspapers of varying degrees of obscurity.

The letter and pamphlet were followed after an interval by another letter, as follows:

Dear Friend,

Referring to your application for my Pamphlet some time back, I shall be glad to know whether you wish me to proceed further in the matter. As I have received no letter from you, I presume that you imagine the cost of treatment will be too high. I will, therefore, make you a Special Offer, that is, for the sum of 10s. (which may be paid in two monthly instalments of 5s. each, if more convenient) I will forward you the full Treatment and Directions. Should you avail yourself of this offer, kindly detach the form at the bottom of this letter and return to me. The Treatment is, without doubt, the most effectual ever placed before the Public, as will be found by the numerous testimonials received.

I am daily in receipt of letters similar to those enclosed herewith, and I feel confident that, should you give the treatment a trial, you will also be able to report quite as good results.

Kindly let me know your decision as soon as possible. If you will take my advice you will not further delay.

May I draw your attention to the letters on the other side?

I am, yours faithfully,

HERBERT CLIFTON.

The "treatment form" was filled up and sent in with 10s., and, as was to be expected, "my candid opinion as to whether my system of treatment is calculated to efficiently meet the requirement," was apparently in favour of treating the case, as a pair of "drum-supports" and a bottle of fluid were received, together with a letter asking the recipient to follow out the directions given very carefully and not be disheartened "because you find no improvement immediately, you must give the Cure a fair trial. I shall be glad," the letter concluded, "to hear from you in about three weeks' time with a general report on your case."

The "drum-supports" consisted of half-inch lengths of narrow india rubber tubing, as used for the valves of bicycle tyres, with an inner tube of "gum-elastic," the india rubber being expanded at one end into a funnel ¼ in. long, and attached at the other to a small oval disc of sheet india-rubber. The prime cost of the pair would probably not exceed 3d. The bottle was labelled "No. 1. Price 3s.," and contained 1 fluid ounce of liquid; analysis showed this to have the following composition:

Glycerine	10 per cent. approx.
Oil	28 ,, ,,
Ether	2 ,, ,,
Water	to 100

A trace (about 0·01 per cent.) of an alkaline substance was present, which appeared to be borax. The oil showed the characters of almond oil.

The estimated cost of the ingredients, for 1 oz., is one halfpenny.

OHRSORB COMPOUND.

The following advertisement is taken from *Cassell's Saturday Journal*:

DOCTOR MAKES DEAF HEAR

A medical book just published describes a German doctor's wonderfully simple cure for deafness and head noises (a real home cure). A limited number of those books have been secured for readers of *Cassell's Saturday Journal*, and will be sent free by post by the publisher, M. Franckel.

Application to the London address given brought a pamphlet of sixteen pages, from which a few extracts are here given:

For years it has been known to Medical Men that the minute vessels or channels of the lymphatic system underlying the skin, covering the bone behind the ear, were intimately connected with those supplying vital nourishment to the middle and internal ear, where we find the common seat of deafness and head noises. If, then, we could medicate through the skin, this important current of lymphatic fluid, controlling the health of the essential parts of the organ of hearing, our medications could be made to flow inward to reach and to cure a disease so deeply hidden within the ear as to be otherwise regarded as incurable. It is the province of this little work to explain why the prescriptions of so many aurists have failed in years past, and to present a new chemical compound which is of the utmost value to deaf people.

Applications behind the ear are recommended in the writings of our greatest ear surgeons. Gruber, Politzer, Delstanche, Grünfeld, and numerous others have given us prescriptions of this kind, and, although their combinations of drugs have failed to produce any remarkable results, they have pointed out the remedies that would cure if combined with a substance which could penetrate the skin freely. . . Until lately we possessed no basis for our ointments, embrocations, or plasters, which could freely penetrate the skin. . . . Happily there is a new basis lately brought to the notice of the medical profession, which has the remarkable property of uniting with the watery secretions of the body in such a way that it (*sic*) absorbed by the skin, and taken up by the lymphatic circulation (described on p. 1), together with any drugs that are combined with it in the form of an ointment. , , To this new basis has been given the name " Ohrsorb."

Quotations purporting to be from the writings of medical men are given, but no references are provided by which they can be checked; and, indeed, the extracts only refer to a "new preparation" and a "new treatment," without any indication that the advertised article is the one intended. Another quotation is then given "From the Private Clinical Memoranda of Dr. Kupfinn," described as an "Hon. Auris Chirurgis," in which "Ohrsorb" is referred to in a laudatory manner; this is followed by an account of some "typical cases," but it does not appear that this is part of the quotation, although it is so put that it might easily be taken to be. The pamphlet continues :

It should be clearly understood that Ohrsorb by itself is only a basis used solely for the purpose of providing the *active portion* of the Author's Absorption Treatment, and that the cure depends on the medicinal action of the drugs compounded with it in any special prescription. It is for this reason that certain particulars as to each patient's case are asked for on the enclosed coupon, namely, that the individual form of deafness, head noises, or ear trouble may be treated by an " Ohrsorb " compound specially adapted to it.

The pamphlet proceeds to give reasons for supplementing the treatment by the use of other articles, of which the following are recommended : " Ohraseptic," " Nazaseptic," " Specially Prepared Catarrh Tonic," a nasal irrigator, and a safety ear syringe. It was accompanied by a leaflet headed, "Medical Report on the 'Ohrsorb' Treatment," in which many testimonials are given, but not one from a medical source or anything of the nature of a medical report; also by a "reduced price coupon," offering a 2s. 9d. tube for 1s. 6d. or a 4s. 6d. tube for 3s., provided the applicant undertook to use it as directed and report the result, and a list of about fifty questions to be answered in connexion with deafness, &c., and catarrh of the nose and throat, concluding with the following paragraph :

As a little return for supplying the tube of "Ohrsorb" compound at the reduced price, and for the very special attention that will be given to your case, the author will be grateful if you favour him with the names and addresses of two or three of your friends who suffer from deafness, head noises, or catarrh of the nose or throat. This is entirely confidential, and your name will not be mentioned.

In order to test the importance attached to the answers to the questions, a supply of "Ohrsorb Compound for Deafness" was sent for, without giving any particulars of the supposed case for which it was required. The compound was at once sent, together with a multiple-typed letter of the usual kind, as shown by the following extracts :

"I hope you will not neglect to write me about your progress with my treatment"; "of course you will appreciate that in obstinate cases Ohrsorb must be persisted with for some time before the improvement can begin to show itself."

and offering for future supplies three 4s. 6d. tubes for 10s. 6d.

The "Special Ohrsorb Compound" is supplied in collapsible tubes, and the 2s. 9d. size contained just over $\frac{1}{2}$ oz. of ointment. The directions were to rub the ointment once, twice, or thrice a day over the skin close behind the ear, and also from just beneath the ear around to the front of the throat, for three to five minutes.

The ointment, nearly black in colour, contained about 70 per cent. of vaseline, and about 4 per cent. of beeswax, a little soap, and a little saponifiable fat ; sulphur and ammonia were present in combination, and the dark constituent appeared to be of the class represented by thiol, tumenol, and petrosulfol, artificial compounds intended to take the place of ichthyol, and like it containing much sulphur in combination but free from its disagreeable odour. The total sulphur found in "Ohrsorb Compound" was 0·8 per cent., which corresponds to about 8 per cent. of one of these substances. An ointment made up with tumenol, soft paraffin, wax, and a little ammonia soap resembled "Ohrsorb Compound" very closely, though the correspondence was not quite complete. It was not considered worth while to isolate the dark constituent in a state of purity permitting of more precise identification than is here indicated; to determine the detailed characterization of such a substance a large quantity would be necessary.

CHAPTER XVI

REMEDIES FOR EYE DISEASES.

THE proprietary articles advertised for the cure of diseases of the eyes, though perhaps not so numerous as some other classes of nostrums, vary a good deal in nature, but the claims made for most of them are equally comprehensive. The results of analysis of a few are here given and it will be seen that two of them, including one called " botanic," are mercurial ointments. Another advertiser seems to think or pretends to think that cataract can be cured by bathing the eyes with soda alum dissolved in coloured water, while we come across also an " Ophthalmic Institution " selling for external application an anti-cataract mixture consisting of glycerine with a little potassium iodide and starch.

SINGLETON'S EYE OINTMENT

This is stated to be prepared, by a person whose name is not Singleton, at an address in London. The price charged is 2s. for a pot containing about 55 grains.

The ointment is described on the outer package as

" An Absolute Specific for all Eye Troubles and Diseases."

On a circular enclosed in the package it was stated:

" It cures Weak Sight, Inflamed Eyes, and all disorders of the Eyelids from whatever cause arising. . . Singleton's Eye Ointment requires great skill in making, and is composed of costly ingredients. One pot will cure you. . . The Ointment also cures Piles and Scorbutic Eruptions."

A book dealing with the ointment was also supplied, in which it is stated that

" Singleton's Eye Ointment will cure all affections of the eye."

Analysis showed the principal ingredient to be red mercuric oxide, of which 7·4 per cent. was present. The fatty basis contained about 4 per cent. of beeswax, and the remainder was a practically neutral and colourless substance which agreed in properties and analytical figures with a mixture of lard, Japan wax, and purified cocoanut oil. It is, of course, impossible to determine with certainty the composition of a mixture of fats, unless a large quantity is available for analysis; but the exact nature of the fatty basis is immaterial, and no indication was obtained of any other medicinal ingredient.

The assertion that such an ointment "requires great skill in making" is absurd, and as to the costliness of the ingredients, the 55 grains in the pot are estimated to be worth one-ninth of a penny.

BOSTOCK'S EYE OINTMENT.

This ointment, stated to be manufactured by a limited company with an address in London, is sold in a pot containing half an ounce, and costing 1s. 1½d. It is described on the label as "An invaluable remedy for every Disease to which the Eye is subject." In a circular wrapped round the pot it is called "Bostock's Botanic Eye Ointment," which

is strongly recommended as a valuable Restorative and Preserver of the Sight, removing Inflammation, Bloodshots, Scorbutic Humours, Shooting Pains, Dimness, Swelling in the Eyelids, and numerous other diseases to which the Eye is subject; it also preserves the Sight against the injuries arising from extreme Heat and Cold.

Analysis showed the presence of small quantities of ammoniated mercury (commonly known as white precipitate) and an insoluble compound of lead which appeared to be the oxide; a little glycerine was present, and a bitter, light-coloured substance of the nature of an extract; this contained no alkaloid, and gave no characteristic reactions indicating the drug or plant from which it was derived; a trace of a vegetable powder was also found, the quantity being so very small that it was probably only an accidental contamination of the extract; when examined microscopically it appeared to consist chiefly of the tissue of a seed. The basis of the ointment contained soft paraffin and spermaceti, and a third constituent agreeing in its characters with lard. Determination of the amounts of the respective ingredients indicated the following approximate formula :

Ammoniated mercury	0·88 per cent.
Lead oxide (litharge)	0·15 ,,
Glycerine	2·25 ,,
Extractive	3·32 ,,
Spermaceti	31·0 ,,
Soft paraffin	31·0 ,,
Lard	31·4 ,,

Neglecting the extractive, the estimated cost of the ingredients for half an ounce is under one halfpenny.

A NEW AND MARVELLOUS REMEDY FOR THE EYES.

This substance, sold from an address in Wisbech at the price of 2s. 9d. for a packet containing 135 grains, was enclosed in a small envelope, on which was written, "Remedy for Eyes only"; there was no printed label except the revenue stamp. In the accompanying circular it was described in the following terms :

A Cure for Cataracts, Films, White Specks, &c. without Operation. The Remedy Cures and Improves the Sight when every other remedy and human skill fails. The Remedy within Twelve Months has proved itself to have no equal for removing Cataracts, Films, White Specks, &c., and is guaranteed the greatest and most marvellous Remedy in the world for such, and for all Eye Sufferers.

Directions for use were given in another circular, as follows, and seem worth quoting as an illustration of pretensions so preposterous that they seem calculated to defeat their own object even when addressed to the most credulous :

Divide the packet of powder into four parts; into an ordinary six ounce medicine bottle put one part out of the four, then fill up the bottle with pure water. Filter or strain the water before so doing, then let the Lotion stand all night after it is made, it is then ready for use. Keep the remainder of the powder in a dry place until required for use.

Shake up the bottle well before using, and in case of Blindness or very bad eyesight, for deep-seated Inflammation, Cataracts, White Specks, &c., pour some of the Lotion into an earthen cup or basin, and bathe the eyes three times a day, about two minutes at a time, and let the Lotion go well into the eyes by winking them whilst bathing them—the Lotion will do no harm by going well into them, for good results can only be obtained in such cases by the remedy going well into the eyes. After bathing the eyes cover up the Lotion with a saucer or plate to keep dust, etc., out, until required for use again. Use a piece of linen rag for bathing the eyes.

N.B.—For Painful, Bloodshot, Weak, Dim, and Misty Eyes, or Floating Black Specks, or for Eye Strain, Etc., and for Strengthening the Optic Nerve, Etc., and for Inflammation, Short Sight, Etc.—Simply bathe the eyes twice a day, morning and night, just before going to bed, about two minutes at a time, letting a little of the Lotion go into the eyes, and should the Remedy make the eyes smart too much, and too long, or make the eyes inflamed or water, etc., too much, make the Remedy a little weaker by adding a little more water to same quantity of Powder, or by not putting quite so much powder to same quantity of water.

This circular concludes with the following notice :

Please Note the Remedy can only be had direct from the Proprietor himself, as no other human being in existence sells it.

The package was accompanied by a written paper as follows :

Please note. Since instructions have been printed I find it necessary for a slight alteration for the benefit of those suffering from Cataracts, Films, and white specks. In such cases when first commencing to use the remedy divide the packet of powder into 4 parts make one bottle out of one part and use according to instructions. After the use of first bottle divide the rest of the powder into 2 parts you will then have sufficient for 2 bottles and will therefore have remedy much stronger of which is needed in case of Cataracts, etc. And when more remedy is required always divide the packet into 3 parts sufficient to make 3 bottles and follow instructions.

(P.S.) I may say for the benefit of those suffering from Cataracts, Films, and white specks the best and quickest results have been obtained by using one bottle per week.

The packet contained a coarse pink powder, with many white particles. Analysis showed it to contain :

Basic aluminium sulphate	48·2 per cent.
Sodium sulphate (anhydrous)	18·3 ,,
Colouring matter	a trace.

the remainder being water. The double sulphate of aluminium and sodium, or soda alum, contains 48·8 per cent. of aluminium sulphate and 20·3 per cent. of sodium sulphate, and the substance under examination thus practically consisted of this salt, somewhat deficient in sulphuric acid. The colouring matter did not quite agree in its behaviour with any of the common pink colours, though it was very similar to acid magenta.

The estimated cost of 135 grains is one-twentieth of a penny.

POMIES' ANTI-CATARACT MIXTURE.

This application is sold from a place called an Ophthalmic Institution in London at the price of 2s. 6d. for a pot containing 162 grains.

It is one of a series of preparations sold under the name "Pomies," including anti-cataract oil, anti-inflammation eye lotions Nos. 1 and 2, sedative collyrium, and others. The package itself was singularly free from printed matter; the directions on the label were as follows:

"Take some of the Mixture on a camelhair brush and introduce it into the eye in wiping the brush between the lids two or three times, twice a day."

Analysis showed the composition of the substance to be:

Potassium iodide	5·6 per cent.
Glycerine	56·5 ,,
Starch	6·4 ,,
Water	31·5 ,,

The estimated cost of the ingredients, for 162 grains, is one-third of a penny.

SOME GERMAN NOSTRUMS.

The eye preparations analysed by Dr. Zernik are not very interesting. One called *Okterin* is a sulphate water, colourless, odourless, acid, and astringent, apparently pumped out of a mine containing ochre. Another sold under the name *Opthalmol*, and described as a natural remedy for all kinds of eye disease is supposed to be made from the glands of a fish. It yielded analytical data which appeared to prove that it was rancid olive oil, with 6 or 7 per cent. of a mineral oil like paraffin. A third wonder-working application, *Augenwol*, said to be made from various plants obtained from many countries proved to be a coloured and perfumed solution of common salt containing a little glycerine and some extractive substances.

CHAPTER XVII.

REMEDIES FOR PILES.

THE series of analyses of secret remedies for haemorrhoids, and the extracts from the advertisements by which these nostrums are commended to the public, make it evident that the prevalence of this complaint, which is always disagreeable and painful, and sometimes incapacitating, provides a happy hunting ground for the nostrum-monger. An additional attraction is, perhaps, to be found in the fact that considerable variety is possible in the method of treatment. Local applications, represented by suppositories and ointments, appear to be most in favour, but there is an obvious opportunity for the man who wishes to sell a medicine to be taken internally to declare that local applications "only afford temporary ease, and do not tend to remove the cause. Only internal treatment can cure." The further possibility of extracting double or threefold payments from sufferers by insisting on the necessity of both local and internal remedies has by no means been neglected; in some cases one preparation only is advertised, and after obtaining this the sufferer learns that something further must be bought if the promised cure is to be effected. In another case, where the remedy is a "threefold treatment, because there are three avenues of approach to the seat of the ailment," it is advertised to be sent without payment, the money to be paid after a week's trial if benefit has been received; any one availing himself of this offer necessarily supplies the vendors with his name and address, and will then, it seems, become the recipient of numerous letters, emphasizing the dangers of neglect, and offering "our full-size guinea treatment" on special terms. It has been shown in previous chapters that this method of doing business directly with the persons taking quack remedies is in great, and apparently growing, favour with makers of such things. The letters with which the sufferer is inundated are, as a rule at any rate, printed in imitation of type-written letters or reproduced by some manifolding process, and the recipient, unless he be something of an expert, is likely to suppose that he is receiving letters composed for his personal benefit, an illusion that is sedulously maintained by a profession of "special interest in your case," or some equivalent fiction. The majority of the preparations described in this chapter contain substances commonly employed for the relief of piles, such as hamamelis (witch hazel), lead acetate, zinc oxide, calomel, or others, if possible, still more old-fashioned; some, like the "Muco-Food Cones, containing concentrated glutinous nourishment," consist of flour and cocoa butter, and are innocent of medicinal ingredients. Advertisers, of course, indulge in the usual impudent reflexions on the work of the medical profession; one, for instance, hazards the statement that "for centuries piles have been treated in a careless, listless, manner by physicians, who, through ignorance or indifference, were unfit to be entrusted with such cases." These same advertisers remark: "The people do not like to be humbugged"—a statement, perhaps, as far from the truth as some other assertions in the advertisements and letters. One company—two of whose "cures" have been shown in previous chapters to consist of sugar only, and whose ointment for piles is about equally active —invites those who are not cured by it to detail their symptoms to "our medical correspondence department"; it is easy to believe that "you will receive the same thorough attention from our medical staff as if you were examined personally," but how much attention that would be is wisely not stated. The majority of the articles are of American origin, some of them being marked "Made in U.S.A.," and others being now prepared in this country, but having originally come from across the Atlantic. Whether English or foreign, however, the usual disproportion is to be found between the prime cost and the price charged. If in the present series the highest price is charged—and the greatest pertinacity in extracting the sufferer's money is shown—by a transatlantic concern, in other chapters English quacks have been shewn well to the fore as regards both price and methods.

BUER'S PILES CURE.

On purchasing from an address in one of the Home Counties Buer's "Piles Cure" for 1s. 1½d., it proved to consist of a box of Buer's Mul'la, and a single sample powder of Buer's Pile Powders, which cost a further 1s. 1½d. for a box. Several circulars were enclosed in the package. The trade-mark was a picture of a donkey; a few extracts will suffice as specimens of the statements made:

Is it money (1s. 1½d.) or your life? Buer, the founder, the proprietor, is the seventh son, not trading on his birthright but on his cure, testified by hundreds. Warrants it will cure you. If you suffer, will you try it?

The pains experienced range all the way from the slightest itch to the most terrible sufferings, which appear like tearing the body asunder, and unless the piles are cured with Buer's Mul'la there is no relief. . .

They cause you to be despondent, caring little to live; no go in you; quarrel. some in yourself; weakening to the constitution; until something gives way and hastens your death. It is therefore money or your life; no hesitation.

But one thing—not for the sake of selling the Powders—keep a box of Buer's Pile Powders in house—12 for 1s. 1½d. ain't dear—and take one as directed whenever you feel any irritation.

The box of ointment contained two-fifths of an ounce. The directions were:

Apply this Mul'la to parts affected.

Analysis showed the ointment to contain:

Lanoline (anhydrous)	66·5 per cent.
Beeswax	1·5 ,,
Water	32·0 ,,

Hamamelis ointment is usually made from the liquid extract which contains rectified spirit, but no alcohol was present in this oddly-named preparation; it may have been made with liquor hamamelidis prepared without the use of alcohol; a minute trace of water-soluble substance contained in the ointment suggested by its behaviour with reagents that such was the case. The estimated cost of ingredients is three farthings.

Twelve of the powders are supplied in the 1s. 1½d. box. The directions are:

To be taken at bedtime in a glass of milk or water.

Analysis showed the composition to be:

Precipitated sulphur	14·9 grains,
Calcined magnesia (partly carbonated)	23·6 ,,

in one powder of average weight. Single powders in one box varied from 28 to 48 grains. The estimated cost of the ingredients for twelve powders is 1¼d.

MUNYON'S PILE OINTMENT.

This ointment is supplied by the same Homoeopathic Home Remedy Company as has been encountered in earlier chapters. The price charged was 1s. a package, containing a collapsible tube holding 1 oz. of ointment and a metal tube for introducing it.

On the outside of the package it was stated that the ointment

permanently cures all forms of Piles or Hemorrhoids, and immediately relieves pain, burning, itching, and distress at the outlet of the bowels.

In the circular enclosed in the package, in which thirty of this company's preparations for different complaints were advertised, it was stated that the ointment

cures piles, blind or bleeding, protruding or internal, stops itching instantly, allays inflammation, and gives ease at once to the sore parts, heals fissures, ulcerations, cracks, and all anal troubles."

A label on the tube of ointment asked the purchaser

if this remedy fails to cure him, to write to the proprietor stating fully all your symptoms. He will have your case carefully diagnosed, and, you will receive the same thorough attention from our medical staff as if you were examined personally. All communications are kept strictly confidential, and replies are sent in plain envelopes. Our Medical Correspondence Department is having great success in curing old obstinate cases. Remember we sweep away all fees for medical advice, we put special medical attention at your service absolutely free. We want you to feel at liberty to write us whenever you need any medical advice, and to fully understand that there will be no charge of any kind for our service.

Analysis showed the ointment, which was directed to be applied three times a day, to consist of soft paraffin, with a trace of ichthyol sufficient to give a slight odour, but not enough to affect the appearance of the ointment. Experiments showed that 0·2 per cent. or over of ichthyol appreciably darkens the colour of soft paraffin, and it appears therefore that less than this proportion was present. The estimated cost of one ounce of the ointment is one farthing.

DOAN'S OINTMENT.

This is sold by a company giving an address in London; the price is 2s. 9d. a tin, containing 1⅔ oz.

On the package it was stated that

Doan's Ointment cures Piles, Salt Rheum, Chilblains, Eczema. Cures Black-headed Pimples, Hives and any itching disease.

In the enclosed circular it was referred to as:

The "Thorough" Cure for Piles, Eczema, Shingles, and Itching Diseases of the Skin.

And the statement was made that:

Bleeding and torturing itching piles are quickly and thoroughly cured by Doan's Ointment, relief being usually obtained from the first application. A cure will follow—a "thorough" cure.

A "Pile Pipe" was supplied at 6d. for applying the ointment to internal piles; for external piles it was directed to be applied with the finger or a piece of clean soft rag. Analysis showed the composition of the ointment to be:

Calomel	36·0 per cent.
Zinc oxide	11·2 ,,
Phenol	1·3 ,,
Beeswax	2·3 ,,
Soft paraffin	49·2 ,,

The estimated cost of the ingredients is 2d.

OXIEN MEDI-CONE PILE TREATMENT.

The sole proprietors of this treatment are stated to be "The Giant Oxie Co.," of a town in the U.S.A., but having a British depôt in London. The price charged for a box was 2s. 3d.; it contained twelve suppositories, described on the label as:

Warranted to cure Blind, Bleeding, or Itching Hemorrhoids, and all other Diseases of the Lower Bowel and Rectum.

The following extracts are quoted from the enclosed circulars:

Just so far as an electric light is ahead of a tallow candle, is the Oxien Medi-Cone Pile Treatment in advance of and superior to all other remedies for Rectal Diseases.

The people do not like to be humbugged. Modern Men and Women demand modern methods of treatment. With this in view we have after careful painstaking study and experimenting organized a radically new method for the positive cure of Bleeding or Itching Piles or Hemorrhoids, Rectal Ulcers, Fissure, Polypi, Fistula, and all ailments of the Rectum and Lower Bowel. . .

If you are a sufferer from this terrible malady which has scourged people of all classes of society, in every clime since Bible times, do not now give up. You can be cured. For centuries Piles have been treated in a careless, listless manner, by physicians who through ignorance or indifference were unfit to be entrusted with such cases, or by quacks who by questionable methods and high-titled nostrums extracted dollar after dollar from patient sufferers. During the past few years, however, a great awakening has taken place. The people demanded a suitable and satisfactory treatment and students have been at work, and the subject and its cures have had the most careful and scientific attention.

The result of the careful and scientific attention of the students is these suppositories, which were found on analysis to have the following composition:

Lead acetate	5·6 per cent.
Creasote, about	2·0 „
A resinoid substance	3·0 „
Vegetable tissue	1·0 „
Hard paraffin	7·0 „
Oil of theobroma (cocoa butter)	81·4 „

The resinoid substance showed the presence of tannin; it could not be identified with any certainty, but may have been "hamamelin," an extract of hamamelis (witch hazel) for which there is no official standard or method of preparation, but it did not agree closely in character with the hamamelin ordinarily supplied in this country. The vegetable tissue appeared to be that of a young leaf, and from the peculiar nature of the hairs was probably hamamelis leaf; the mature leaves as imported into Great Britain, however, possess characters which were absent. The suppositories were of the average weight of 19 grains, and the estimated prime cost of the ingredients for twelve is 1¼d.

HEMOTORA.

The fluid to which this name is given is stated to be manufactured for a company by a chemist in Cheshire. A bottle containing nearly 4 fluid ounces, costs 2s. In the accompanying circular the company's views as to the cause of piles are expounded as follows:

> Hemotora-is a Concentrated Extract of Herbs which has been tested and proved beyond doubt to be a " Certain Specific for Piles." A short explanation will clearly show the action of Hemotora. Should any hindrance occur to the flow of blood through the hæmorrhoidal veins, they naturally become congested and distended; this further brings about a thickening of the vein walls, eventually developing painful tumours called " Piles," or technically, " Hæmorrhoids." The many and various conditions that eventually produce Piles can always be traced to this accumulation of blood, and it is in this direction, the very basis of the complaint, that the active principles of Hemotora display their wonderful efficiency by removing the obstruction to the natural flow of blood; the parts will then return to their original condition and functions. Relief may be obtained from the external use of Ointments, Creams and Suppositories, but these preparations only afford temporary ease, and do not tend to remove the Cause. Only internal treatment can cure. Results show that External, Internal, and Bleeding Piles alike soon yield to this remedy; after a few doses the pain is greatly alleviated, accompanied by a sense of relief from the sickly feeling of lassitude and depression. The tonic properties of Hemotora quickly restore the general health.

From another circular it appears that

> The "Hemotora Salve" for Itching Piles is sold in small 1s. Jars, large size, 2s. 6d.

Analysis of "Hemotora" showed it to be an aqueous liquid containing about 0·09 per cent. of a bitter amorphous alkaloid and 2·7 per cent of vegetable extractive, including a little of a substance of the nature of a tannin, but not medicinal tannic acid. The liquid appeared to be produced by aqueous extraction, infusion or decoction, of some bitter vegetable substance.

ROLLO'S REMEDY FOR PILES.

This ointment, made by a Scottish company, is sold in tins, price 1s. 1½d., containing rather under 1 oz. It is described in an accompanying circular as a remedy for a good many disorders besides Piles:

> Rollo's Remedy for Piles, Eczema, Rheumatic Pains, Burns and Scalds, Chilblains, Soreness or Roughness of the Skin, Itching.

Rollo's Remedy is a Vegetable Extract in the Highest Possible State of Purity, without any addition whatever. It is obtained from a little known part of Africa, and has been brought to its present perfection after a long series of scientific experiments. It does not contain any Poisons, Drugs, Chemicals, or Impurities of any kind, and although intended for external use only, it is so pure that even if eaten it would be quite harmless.

Analysis showed the ointment to contain over 99 per cent. of fatty basis, with a very small quantity of a dark substance which appeared to be vegetable extractive. It contained no alkaloid and no tannin, and possessed no characters indicative of the drug or plant from which it was derived. The basis showed the characters of a mixture of fats in which oil of theobroma (cocoa butter) predominated, with about 15 per cent. of lanoline (anhydrous).

DR. VAN VLECK'S COMPLETE ABSORPTIVE PILE TREATMENT.

The preparations sold under this name are, or were, very widely advertised by a company giving an address in London. They are offered without previous payment, as indicated by the following extracts from an advertisement:

To every person who sends us the coupon below at once, we will send— Free to try—our complete new threefold absorption cure for Piles, Ulcer, Fissure, Prolapse, Tumours, Constipation, and all rectal troubles. If you are fully satisfied with the benefits received, send us 4s. 6d. If not, we take your word, and it costs you nothing; you decide after a thorough trial.

Our valuable new Pile Book (in colours) comes free with the approval treatment all in plain package. Send no money—just the coupon—to Dr. Van Vleck Co.

The "new Pile Book," a pamphlet of 40 pages, entitled "The Rational Treatment of Rectal Diseases," included a description of the rectum, with eleven illustrations—several of them coloured —with descriptions of various kinds of piles and treatments, and of the Van Vleck remedies. A few extracts only can be given:

Unless you are beyond every chance of recovery, this wonderful threefold Absorption treatment will cure you. . .

The Absorption Cure is Threefold because there are three avenues of approach to the seat of the ailment. To neglect one of these avenues means to leave an open gateway for the return of the malady. Dr. Van Vleck struck at the well spring of the disease, as well as at the visible effect of it. Once cured

by our treatment the disease is cured to stay cured. 'There is no pain, no confinement, no heavy doctor's or surgeon's bill, no operation. The cost is placed within the reach of all, and the treatment is accompanied by a positive guarantee of cure. The treatment embraces:
1. Dr. Van Vleck's Absorptive Plasma.
2. Dr. Van Vleck's Muco-food Cones.
3. Dr. Van Vleck's Pile Pills (and System Regulator).

The "positive guarantee" is given inside the back cover of the pamphlet, as follows:

GUARANTEE.

The Dr. Van Vleck Co. . . . Hereby positively agrees that Dr. Van Vleck's Absorption Cure for Piles, when taken and used in accordance with our simple instructions and directions, will cure any case of Piles, and in the event of its failure to cure,

AGREES TO REFUND

The entire amount paid immediately upon required statement that benefit has not been received.   The Dr. Van Vleck Co.

It will be observed that this purported to be a guarantee to cure, and would be read by most as a promise to refund the amount paid if the treatment did not cure; whereas it was only a promise to refund if a "required" statement were made that benefit (that is, any benefit) had not been received, a statement most uncured persons might hesitate to make.

On application for the 4s. 6d. treatment, 5 suppositories, 10 pills, and about 65 grains of "plasma" in a collapsible tube were sent, with a long circular letter of the usual type, offering the :

Large special treatment, including our new Rectal Applicator, made from pure Stannum,* for 21s., or for 16s. 6d. in addition to the 4s. 6d. to be sent for what was supplied.

The labels of the preparations were stamped "made in U.S.A."

Letters subsequently received urging continued use of the treatment and pressing for particulars of the case, were much like those from other nostrum dealers which have been printed in earlier chapters, and included such statements as :

We have made a special study of your case, and we are convinced that if this, our final offer to *you*, is accepted, a permanent cure will be assured.

---

* *Stannum* : tin. *Latin Dictionary.*

No "case" had been even mentioned in sending for the preparations. The "final offer" was:

On receipt of 12s. 6d. we will forward you our Full Size Guinea Treatment, post free. We are perfectly willing to trust to you to remit us the balance of 4s. on completion of the cure. Remember you are absolutely protected by our guarantee (see last page of booklet).

Other papers sent were a "Patient's Special Symptom Form," to be filled up after using the "treatment," and including such questions as "Are your Piles better?" "Please state in what way your condition has changed since you commenced taking our treatment," and a form for names and addresses of other persons suffering from piles.

Analysis of the "plasma" showed it to be a paraffin ointment containing about 6 per cent. of powdered galls and a small quantity of menthol (approximately 1 per cent.); the basis consisted principally of soft paraffin, with a dark substance which appeared to be the natural impurities of crude petroleum. The formula is thus approximately:

Powdered galls	6 parts.
Menthol	1 ,,
Crude petroleum jelly to	100 ,,

The "Muco-food Cones" had an average weight of 21 grains; analysis showed them to consist of:

Wheat flour	28 per cent.
Oil of theobroma (cocoa butter)	68 ,,
Water	4 ,,

Careful search failed to show any other ingredient.

The pills were coated with a mixture of talc and sugar, tinted an orange colour; after removing the coating they had an average weight of 1·1 grain. Analysis showed them to contain small quantities of powdered capsicum, powdered liquorice, and maize starch; 23 per cent. of ash, about half of which consisted of silicious matter and was apparently talc that had got into the pill from the coating; the remainder of the ash showed the usual constituents of the ash of vegetable drugs and extracts, together with a small quantity of zinc, which was present in the pill in the metallic state and was presumably derived from some vessel used in the preparation; a bitter extract, agreeing in its properties with extract of cascara sagrada, constituting the major portion of the pill; and a resinoid substance which resembled iridin. As a definite formula cannot be given for such a pill, the cost of ingredients can only be estimated somewhat roughly. After making liberal allowance for the unknown resinoid, the estimated cost of the ingredients of the quantities of the three preparations supplied for 4s. 6d. is three-farthings.

CHAPTER XVIII.

PREPARATIONS FOR RUPTURE.

ADVERTISEMENTS of means of curing rupture without operation are very common, but in most cases the advertiser has for sale a special form of truss or other appliance. The disorder is so well-known to be of a mechanical or structural nature, that it might have been thought that it would hardly have been worth anybody's while to advertise drugs for its cure. Nevertheless there are, at least, two instances in which medicine for internal or external use is supplied; the results of examination of these are here given.

RICE'S TREATMENT FOR RUPTURE.

The following is a specimen of the wording of the advertisement of this " treatment " which used to be, and perhaps still is, very commonly illustrated by a picture of a bricklayer filling up a hole in a wall:

RUPTURE CURED.
Do You See this Bricklayer Closing up the Opening in that Wall. That is the way to cure *Rupture*, by filling in the opening with *new* and *stronger* tissue.

A rupture is simply a break in a wall—the wall of *muscle* that protects the bowels and other internal organs.

It is just as easy to cure a wound or break in *this* muscle as one in the arm or hand.

Now this break may be no larger than the tip of your finger. But it is large *enough* to allow part of the intestines to crowd through. Of course, this cannot *heal* unless nature is *assisted*. That is just what this Method does. It enables you to retain the protrusion inside the wall in its proper place.

Then we give you a Developing Lymphol to apply on the rupture opening. This penetrates *through* the skin to the edges of the opening and removes the *hard ring* which has formed around the break.

Then the *healing* process begins. Nature, no longer handicapped by the protruding bowel and hardened ring at the opening, and stimulated by the action of the Lymphol, throws out *her* supply of lymph, and the opening is again filled with *new muscle*.

Isn't this simple ? Isn't it *reasonable ?* * * *

Simply *write* us and we will post you a *free sample treatment of* the Developing Lymphol and a finely illustrated book on The Nature and Cure of Rupture. Do *not* send any money. Just your *name* and *address* on this Coupon.

Application for particulars of the method of cure brought a book of 40 pages, entitled "The Nature and Cure of Rupture," with a letter, directions for measurement, and other papers. It would seem that if the applicant does not at once become a customer, other letters and booklets are sent at intervals. The titles of some of these booklets which are before us are : " First Aid to the Ruptured," " The Value of a Cure," " A Fireside Reverie," " Facts and Faces," " The Story of Christopher Columbus," and "The Man Who Wondered Why." However much the matter varies, it always leads to the subject of the cure of rupture by Rice's Treatment. The treatment consists of the wearing of an " Appliance " (occasionally referred to as " my perfect truss ") and the application of " Developing Lymphol." The respective parts stated to be played by these are indicated by the following extracts from some of the pamphlets referred to :

> To be cured of rupture it is necessary to apply my Lymphol Developing Treatment regularly as directed, for it is the Lymphol, not the Appliance, that performs the cure.
>
> The Appliance is simply a means of support to retain the rupture, and prevent the protrusion from tearing down the new particles of tissue with which the opening is being filled under the vitalizing and healing influence of the Lymphol.

The appliance is supplied in two grades or qualities. The price of the Appliance and Lymphol together ranged from 21s. for a child's single appliance of the cheaper grade to £4 10s. for an " Abdominal Supporter and Navel Appliance Combined," of the higher grade. It was stated in the price list that the lymphol and appliance were not supplied separately; but in another list sent with the goods the lymphol alone was priced at 16s. 6d. The bottle sent held just over four fluid ounces.

The directions were :

> Lie on your back, remove appliance, unscrew stopper, and sprinkle a few drops of the Lymphol on to the point where the rupture leaves the cavity of the abdomen. Apply night and morning, rubbing in thoroughly with fingers.

If irritation is produced, use less Lymphol, or discontinue its use for a few days. The Lymphol may be reduced in strength by adding Spiritus Rectificatus which can be obtained from any chemist.

The "appliance" consisted of an elastic band to go round the body, fitted with an adjustable pad and an understrap. Analysis showed the "lymphol" to be an alcoholic solution containing essential oils and capsicum resin, and a trace of red colouring matter. Oils of origanum (thyme), peppermint, and spearmint were recognized; the proportion of capsicum was estimated by determining the total solid matter, and by comparing the pungency of dilutions of the lymphol with dilutions of the solutions prepared in imitation; the red colouring matter was not cochineal, or one of the common vegetable colours, but appeared to be one of the artificial dyes. Careful comparisons indicated the following formula:

Tincture of capsicum (B.P. strength but prepared with strong alcohol)	60 parts by measure.
Oil of origanum	6 ,, ,,
Oil of peppermint....	1 ,, ,,
Oil of spearmint	0·3 ,, ,,
Red dye	q.s. ,, ,,
Rectified spirit to	100 ,, ,,

The estimated cost of the ingredients for 4 fluid ounces is 9d.

HEALINE TREATMENT.

This is advertised from a town in the south of England as follows:

Rupture cured
speedily and permanently, with inexpensive home treatment. A certain remedy for Man, Woman, and Child. Full particulars on receipt of two stamps.

Application to the address given brought a booklet of 28 pages, headed:

The following is a description of
Rupture,
Its causes, Symptoms,
Treatment, and Cure.

An extract from this booklet is here given.

The only possible way to effect a permanent cure is by taking a remedy that will fortify and strengthen the weakened vessels, and so enable them to bear an ordinary strain without injuring them. HEALINE TREATMENT No. 1

has been found by experience to perform this operation after all other so-called treatments have failed. External treatment cannot cure you, for the cause is internal; therefore to effect a cure the cause must be removed. By taking this remedy as directed, a cure may be expected from two to four months, according to description of complaint and length of time affected. From six to nine bottles of this preparation is generally sufficient to effect a cure, or the same quantity of pills. I do not guarantee to completely cure every case, but it will do as much good as nature will allow, and prevent strangulation in every case. I find, after a few years' experience with this remedy, that it is able to absolutely cure ninety out of every hundred cases of rupture, where nine to a dozen bottles have been taken.

Other sections of the pamphlet are devoted to varicocele and varicose veins, for which it appears that "Healine No. 2" and "Healine No. 3" respectively are recommended.

The prices of the preparations (post free) were thus given:

Liquid Form.—3s. per bottle; Three for 8s. 9d.; or Six prepared bottles for 15s.

Pill Form (recommended).—2s. 9d. per box; Three for 8s.; or Six for 13s. 9d.

Healine Lotion (same price as Internal Healine) is always necessary for bad Ulcerated Legs and open or deep-seated Wounds, and never fails to cure when used as directed.

Consultation by appointment only, for which a fee of 2s. 6d. will be charged.

An application for a bottle of liquid "Healine No. 1," with a remittance of 3s., brought in return a box of the pills, with an intimation that these were recommended in preference. The box contained 60 pills, two to be taken three times a day.

The pills were coated with talc, after removal of which they had an average weight of 4 grains. No metallic salts were present, and no alkaloid; about 1 per cent. of an oily liquid of acid nature, apparently oleic acid, was found; small quantities of a tannin, gum, and phlobaphene, a decomposition product of tannin, were present, and a bitter substance which showed no characters by which it could be identified; aloin and extract of cascara sagrada were absent, and all resinous substances, unless in minute quantity; the pill consisted chiefly of indefinite extractive, with about 20 per cent. of a vegetable powder, one ingredient of which was liquorice, a second appearing to be gentian, but it was not identified with certainty; a considerable portion of the vegetable powder had no identifiable properties.

CHAPTER XIX.
CURES FOR INEBRIETY.

For a good many years past cures for inebriety have been freely advertised in various ways, some of them commonplace and others showing a good deal of ingenuity. Some are advertised and sold in the same way as ordinary secret remedies, that is to say, the purchaser sends so much money and receives a box or bottle with directions for administering the contents. In other instances the inebriate is required to submit himself to inspection, and in certain cases must enter a home maintained by the proprietor or his agents. Between these two extremes there are intermediate plans, the methods followed shading off on the one hand into those of the ordinary nostrum seller, and on the other into the more elaborate system of the "treatments" with which transatlantic enterprise has made us familiar. The last of the remedies described by name below approximates very closely to this class.

COZA POWDER.

This powder is supplied by the Coza Institute, 76, Wardour Street, London, W., formerly 62, Chancery Lane, London, W.C. The price charged for a box, containing 30 powders was 10s.

The preparation was advertised with an offer of a free sample. An application for a sample brought a single powder together with a 10s. box to be paid for or returned, a book of 130 pages (which is referred to below), and a letter, from which the following is an extract:

Coza Powder has the marvellous effect of producing a repugnance to intoxicating drink of any kind, and may be administered in coffee, tea, milk, water, beer, whisky, brandy, or solid food without the partaker's knowledge.

Coza Powder does its work so silently and surely that any person interested in the intemperate can administer it to him or her without his or her knowledge and without him or her learning what has effected the reformation.

Coza Powder has reconciled thousands of families, saved from shame and dishonour thousands of men and transformed them into sturdy citizens and capable business men. It has led many a young man along the direct road to good fortune, and has prolonged by several years the lives of many individuals.

We particularly wish to draw your attention to the fact that we guarantee Coza Powder to be absolutely harmless.

The book which was sent, entitled *No more Drunkenness*, opens with the statements that—

Coza Powder is one of the greatest discoveries of the day. There is nothing in the whole world to compare with it. It is the only powder to cure the craving for drink and drug habits.

The first few pages are devoted to a disquisition on drunkenness; then follow further claims for Coza Powder, such as—

Coza is the name of a marvellous powder which possesses the quality of occasioning in him who takes it a dislike for alcoholic liquors and all intoxicating drinks. The drinker finds alcohol so detestable that even on the most tempting occasions it will be impossible for him to take a single drop.

A large part of the book is given up to what are called testimonials, with portraits stated to represent the writers; the large majority of these are dated from Continental countries. Those to which English names and addresses are appended are for the most part expressions of hopefulness, or records of slight variations in drinking which are believed to be due to the powders; for instance:

My friend has been taking " Coza " this last two days, and he has had no desire for drink.

Enclosed you will find P.O. for which send me another box. I think the powders are doing my friend good. Send at once.

The last pages of the book are devoted to advertisements of Canexia Hair Elixir, Canexia-Brilliantine, and Canexia-Shampoo Powder, supplied from the Canexia Chemical Works, 61, Chancery Lane; and Anticelta Tablets for Obesity, and Brixa Tablets for Thin People, supplied from 62, Chancery Lane.

A visit to the address showed that the Canexia Chemical Works, the Coza Institute, and the offices of Anticelta and Brixa Tablets were all at that time accommodated in three rooms on the second floor at 61 and 62, Chancery Lane, the double number representing the one entrance of a large block of buildings containing hundreds of different offices. A photograph of the entire block, inscribed " Coza Institute," is given in the book just referred to. The address has since been changed to that given above.

The powders had an average weight of 1½ grains, the weights of single ones varying from ⅓ grain to 3 grains. Analysis showed them to contain 90·5 per cent. of sodium bicarbonate, the remainder being a vegetable powder; microscopic examination of this powder showed that it agreed in all its characters with a mixture of equal parts of cummin fruit and cinnamon. No alkaloid was present, and no other ingredient of any kind could be detected. The formula is thus :

Sodium bicarbonate	90 parts.
Powdered cinnamon	5 ,,
Powdered cummin	5 ,,

Cummin fruit (seeds) have a bitter aromatic taste and a peculiar strong heavy odour. Owing to its disagreeable taste and odour cummin is seldom used in medicine, any medicinal properties it possesses being the same as those of other aromatic and less nauseous umbelliferous fruits.

The estimated cost of the ingredients for 30 powders was one-thirtieth of a penny.

DIPSOCURE.

This nostrum is prepared by a " Chemical Co.," giving an address in Birmingham. The price charged for a box, containing 50 powders, 25 being white and 25 tinted reddish-buff, was 9s.

This article, like the preceding, is advertised with an offer of a free sample. Application for a sample brought also a stream of letters at short intervals, with abundant printed matter. A few extracts from the letters are here given :

Eminent medical men have over and over again declared that if a cure for drunkenness could be discovered both TASTELESS AND ODOURLESS, and placed in the hands of a devoted woman to administer SECRETLY, the greatest difficulty in effecting cures would have been overcome. " Dipsocure " IS TASTELESS and ODOURLESS, and CAN BE administered SECRETLY ; so that it has been our privilege and good fortune to have solved the problem. Whilst counteracting and freeing the alcoholic-laden system of the poison, it is soothing to the nerves and restores the health, and is harmless to the most delicate person.

. . . when a cure has been effected we ask you kindly to acquaint us of the fact, and perhaps you will then consider our agency proposal, showing how a good income can be made by introducing the cure to others. To show you the ease with which it can be sold, if you remit us 10s. three packages will be sent, two of which you can readily dispose of to other sufferers at 9s. each, thus making 8s. profit and obtaining one packet quite free.

The directions for use were:

Give one powder three times a day, before meals, dissolved in half a tea-cup of Hot Coffee, Tea, Whisky, Milk, Gin, &c.

Use either the brown or white powder, as the colour of the liquid may require.

The powders had an average weight of 4·2 grains, single powders varying from 2·9 to 6·0 grains. The composition of both kinds was found to be the same except for the trace of colouring matter contained in the tinted powder. Analysis showed the composition to be—

Acetanilide	6 parts.
Potassium bromide	35 ,,
Sugar of milk	59 ,,

The estimated cost of the ingredients for 50 powders was one-third of a penny.

ANTIDIPSO.

This is supplied by another "Chemical Company," giving an address in London. The price of a box, containing 48 powders, 24 being white, and 24 tinted pinkish-buff, was 10s.

The statements made about this article, in circulars and letters, were very similar to those made about the preceding one. A few extracts will suffice:

You will not forget that to insure an absolute complete and permanent cure for the craving, two boxes are invariably required. We have had data of cures effected with one box, but to make absolutely sure you will do well to immediately send us remittance, to the same value as the last, and get the second box of the specific. Antidipso may be administered with or without the knowledge of the patient. . . We enclose you a booklet showing our agency terms. Kindly give it your attention, as we are confident you will be so surprised and satisfied at the cure which will be effected that you will either yourself want to take up agency with us, or get some one in your district to do so.

The directions were:

Give one powder, dissolved in half a tea-cup of hot coffee, whisky, milk, gin, &c. (using either Brown or White Powder as colour of liquid may require) 3 times a day before meals.

The powders had an average weight of 5·3 grains, single powders ranging from 3·7 to 9·9 grains. The white and tinted powders were made of the same constituents, with a trace of colouring matter added in the latter case, but in different proportions. Analysis showed the composition to be:

WHITE POWDERS.

Potassium bromide	24·5 parts.
Sugar of milk	75·5 ,,

COLOURED POWDERS.

Potassium bromide	35 parts.
Sugar of milk	65 ,,

The estimated cost of the ingredients for 48 powders was one-third of a penny.

THE TEETOLIA TREATMENT.

The following is an extract from an advertisement of a "Teetolia Treatment Association," giving an address in London:

> After years of Drink and Drug taking—
> Cured in 4 days.
> . . . The Teetolia treatment acts so rapidly and so efficiently that within four days from the commencement of administration the insistent craving for drink is absolutely destroyed—so much so, that even the thought of alcohol becomes nauseating. . . Thousands have been cured by this treatment, and we guarantee to cure you. If you write to-day, ... you will receive by return of post a private consultation sheet, together with a valuable book on this subject, post free in plain envelope, and you will be a free man within a week.

On application being made for further particulars, a booklet of twenty pages, entitled *The Teetolia Treatment for Alcoholic Excess, Drug Habits, and Resultant Nervous Diseases*, was sent, together with a letter and a form to be filled up with particulars of the case to be treated. The following are extracts from the booklet:

> The discovery of the Teetolia method and treatment for the permanent eradication of the crave for drink and drugs marks an era in medical science. It is the outcome of a life's study of the subject by one of our best known West End physicians.
> You can, whilst undergoing the treatment, pursue your ordinary methods of living. You continue to take your daily modicum of alcohol; but somehow about the third or fourth day of treatment, without having made any physical or mental effort, you feel that you no longer want a drink; it holds out no attractions to you; its magnetic influence has gone. . . . .
> We are willing to supply you with sufficient medicine for eight days' treatment free of all charge. This will enable you to determine whether the treatment is acting successfully, for at the end of the fourth day an obvious and perceptible

effect should be experienced. We impose no condition; we rely on your candour, honesty, and gratitude that at the end of the eight days' treatment, if you are convinced of the value of the Teetolia Treatment, you will forward to us the ordinary fee—£1 1s.—for same, but if you have derived no benefit from the treatment at the end of the same period, then you are under no obligation whatever to pay us one single penny.

The letters were on headed paper, at the top of which was printed, " All communications strictly confidential," and " Consultations with Physician by appointment." The first letter concluded as follows :

Please therefore fill in and return without delay the special statement sheet and upon our receiving it the Physician will go carefully into the case and will prescribe special medicine, which will reach you with expert advice in the course of two or three days in a perfectly plain sealed package.

The "expert advice," in a letter purporting to be from "The Medical Superintendent," sent with the medicine, contained these passages :

I want, if possible, the patient to use his own endeavours to try and keep off alcohol during the first few days of treatment; if this cannot be done, then the treatment must be commenced when the patient is not drinking, in order to give the medicine a better hold on the system. The dislike for alcohol, which we claim, does not come on all at once.

The eight days' treatment is enough to show you that it will do good, but not sufficient in this case to effect a permanent cure. I would advise the patient to continue for at least a month to six weeks.

This is somewhat widely at variance with the statements quoted above. "You continue to take your daily modicum of alcohol" and " you will be a free man within a week."

The one-guinea "treatment" consisted of $2\frac{1}{6}$ fluid ounces of a liquid of the nature of a vegetable fluid extract.

The directions were :

Half a teaspoonful to be taken in a little water every four hours during the day at 10, 2, 6, and 10 o'c.

Analysis showed this to contain 29·3 per cent. by volume of alcohol and 2·3 per cent. of alkaloid, which consisted principally of quinine. The liquid agreed generally with a diluted liquid extract of cinchona; the amount of alkaloid was just under half what is contained in the official liquid extract of cinchona. Treatment with suitable solvents extracted a trace of a non-alkaloidal bitter substance resembling the bitter substances obtainable from quassia, chiretta, &c.; a preparation of chiretta appeared to be the more probable. No strychnine was present, and no evidence was obtained of any other ingredient.

SOME OTHER DRUG CURES FOR INEBRIETY.

A somewhat frequent constituent of preparations for the treatment of inebriety is atropine, while other preparations contain one or more of the alkaloids belonging to the same group, usually known as the solanaceous alkaloids from the fact that they are all derived from plants of the nat. ord. *Solanaceae*. These alkaloids closely resemble each other in their chemical nature and in their pharmacological properties; the principal members of the group are:

Atropine, $C_{17}H_{23}NO_3$, obtained chiefly from *Atropa belladonna* (deadly nightshade) and *Scopola carniolica*.

Hyoscyamine, $C_{17}H_{23}NO_3$, obtained chiefly from *Hyoscyamus niger* (henbane) and *Scopola* species.

Hyoscine, or scopolamine, $C_{17}H_{21}NO_4$, obtained chiefly from *Scopola* species, *Hyoscyamus niger*, and *Datura alba*.

The two following were originally described as separate substances, but have more recently been shown to consist of mixtures:

Duboisine, obtained from *Duboisia myoporoides*, consists chiefly of hyoscyamine and hyoscine.

Daturine, from *Datura stramonium* (thornapple) consists chiefly of hyoscyamine, with a variable proportion of atropine.

A certain preparation for inebriety is said to contain "stramonine"; as no alkaloid has been described and characterized under this name, it is probably only a variant of daturine, which, as has been said, consists of a natural mixture of hyoscyamine and atropine.

To the above may be added the artificial alkaloid homatropine ($C_{10}H_{21}NO_3$), which has not been found in a plant, but is prepared synthetically; in chemical constitution it is mandelyl-tropeine, atropine being tropyltropeine.

The differences in the action of the four principal solanaceous alkaloids are briefly as follows:

Atropine has a stimulant action on the central nervous system especially on the motor area; it depresses and in large doses paralyses the nerve endings of secretory glands, plain muscle, and the heart.

Hyoscyamine is intermediate in its action between atropine and hyoscine; causes less stimulation of the central nervous system than atropine, and is a weaker sedative and hypnotic than hyoscine. It has the same action peripherally as atropine but is twice as powerful.

Hyoscine resembles atropine in its paralysing effect upon peripheral nerve endings, the action being quicker, more powerful, and less lasting. It does not possess the stimulating effect of atropine upon the brain; depression of the motor area is marked from the first.

Homatropine resembles atropine in its action but is less powerful.

CHAPTER XX.

CURE ALLS.

THE greater number of the proprietary medicines described in these pages are advertised as cures for a wide range of ailments, but usually there is some one disease for the treatment of which they are particularly recommended, so that it has been possible to classify them according to their alleged purposes. In very many other cases, however, the claims made are so wide that the article is put forward as a sort of cure-all. Thus one of the articles described is stated to cure such different disorders as constipation, rheumatism, St. Vitus's dance, heart disease, rickets, sleeplessness, kidney complaints, and women's special ailments, among many others, and is said to be " a real elixir of life in solid form "; the facts as to its composition, ascertained by analysis, show what the possibility of its being a " cure "—for heart disease, for instance—is. As to " Pink Pills," another of the nostrums analysed, which probably owes its popularity partly to bold advertisement and partly to its alliterative name, the method followed appears to be to recommend them for different diseases in different advertisements; personal testimony, or what is put forward as such, from sufferers who have been cured, is made the basis of most of these, and illustrations are employed to catch the eye of the casual reader. Analysis showed that these pills were practically the ordinary iron-carbonate pills commonly called Blaud's pill, which ought to be freshly made. The Pink Pills are of lower strength than usually prescribed, and to judge by the proportion of iron that was found to be in the higher state of oxidation, very carelessly prepared. They differ vastly, however, from other Blaud's pills in the price charged for them. Thus the proprietary Pink Pills are sold at a little over a penny each, while coated Blaud's pills can be bought retail at a few pence a gross, and wholesale in large quantities at a little over a penny a gross. The analyses of other proprietary preparations show a similar disparity between the market price of the drug supplied and the price charged to the person who is beguiled into purchasing; thus thirteen-pence-halfpenny, two shillings and sixpence, and two shillings and ninepence are the selling prices of nostrums, the ingredients of which are estimated to cost respectively one eighth, one-third, and one-tenth of a penny.

Preparations of this class are not in all cases very clearly marked off from those recommended for some special disease, such as have been dealt with in previous chapters, for many of them are recommended for some one disease, of which nearly all others are asserted to be variations.

DR. MARTIN'S MIRACLETTS.

These wonders are supplied by a Medicine Co., from an address in London. The prices are 1s. 1½d., 2s. 9d., 4s. 6d., and 11s. per bottle. A 2s. 9d. bottle contained sixty tablets.

They are described on the package as :

A real Elixir of Life in solid form. The world's greatest remedy.
Cures Constipation, Indigestion, Headache, Neuralgia, Anæmia, Nervous Disorders, Liver Troubles, Rheumatism, Sciatica, Gout, St. Vitus' Dance, Hysteria, Rickets, Heart Disease, Kidney Complaints.
Cures Melancholia, Loss of Appetite, Sleeplessness, Lassitude, Mental Depression, Brain Fag, Palpitation, Stomach Disorders, Women's Special Ailments and Irregularity of Health, etc., etc.

A little book, entitled "A Fortune for All," enclosed in the package, contained the following statements :

Whatever you may be suffering from do not worry or fear, as Dr. MARTIN'S MIRACLETTS will be certain to cure you !
Dr. Martin's Miracletts make the weak and sickly become strong and healthy, and the aged become youthful and full of energy; the tired worn-out look being replaced by an appearance of cheerfulness and vivid health. The pale

and wrinkled face with bad complexion gives way to rosy cheeks and a clear skin; the thin gain flesh, and the stout lose superfluous fat; indigestion quickly disappears, the appetite returns, and a *new life* is open to all.

A separate small slip enclosed in the package was worded as follows:

GUARANTEE.

Dr. Martin's Medicine Company being absolutely confident of the marvellous curative properties of their Miracletts, will willingly refund the money to any purchaser who has taken eighteen Miracletts according to directions, and is not satisfied with the results.

Much less conspicuously, on another slip chiefly devoted to the relative quantities in the packages of different size, it was stated:

Those whose ailments have been of long standing must not expect immediate perceptible results, but with a little patience and perseverance the result is SURE.

The "Miracletts" consisted of sugar-coated tablets, the coating being coloured brown with ferric oxide (so-called chocolate coating). After removal of the coating they had an average weight of 4·3 grains; this included the weight of a strong coating of varnish, which was not removed with the sugar-coating. Analysis showed them to contain valerianates of quinine and zinc, iron oxide, menthol, kaolin in considerable quantity, and a little talc. A substance of extract nature was also present to the extent of about 5 per cent.; It possessed no characteristic taste or other property by which it could be identified; a resinous substance, which was found in small quantity, appeared to be merely the varnish with which the tablets were covered. The quantities of the different ingredients were determined as nearly as possible, and the results indicated the following amounts:

Quinine valerianate	0·4 grain.
Zinc valerianate	0·1 ,,
Ferric oxide	0·3 ,,
Menthol	0·03 ,,
Kaolin and talc	2·3 grains.
In one tablet.	

The estimated cost of the ingredients of the tablets is 4d. a hundred.

THERAPION.

Another "medicine company," also with an address in London, advertises three preparations which it calls Therapion. Therapion

No. 1 was described as "the most efficacious remedy" for "all discharges"; Therapion No. 2 as "the great remedy for impurity of the blood, scurvy, pimples, spots, blotches, pains and swellings of the joints, gout," and so on; and No. 3 as a new French remedy, by the use of which the shattered health will be restored.

The Expiring Lamp of Life Lighted Up Afresh,

and a new existence imparted in place of what had so lately seemed worn, "used up," and valueless. This wonderful medicine is suitable for all ages, constitutions, and conditions, in either sex, and it is difficult to imagine a case of disease or derangement, whose main features are those of debility, that will not be speedily and permanently benefited by this never-failing recuperative essence, which is destined to cast into oblivion everything that had preceded it, for this widespread and numerous class of human ailments.

The claims for No. 3 being so inclusive, it was deemed sufficient to analyse it only. The dose of all three was stated to be the same—a piece about the size of a small marble three or four times a day; as the package, costing 2s. 9d., contained 1¼ oz., and as it was referred to as providing twenty ordinary doses, a single dose would be about 30 grains. The substance consisted of a dark stiff paste smelling strongly of camphor. Analysis showed it to contain, in addition to camphor, glycerine, powdered liquorice, a bitter extract agreeing in all respects with extract of gentian, calcium glycerophosphate, and a trace of alkaloid; there also appeared to be a second extract present. The alkaloid, which amounted to 0·06 per cent. only, could not be identified with any of the ordinary medicinal alkaloids. There was some evidence that the second extract was that of damiana, and a paste made up with this and the other ingredients agreed well with the original; but extract of damiana possesses no distinctive characters by which it can be identified in a mixture. Quantitative determinations were made of those ingredients capable of it, and the proportions of the others estimated by comparison. The results indicated the following formula:

Camphor	2·5 parts.
Glycerine	24 ,,
Powdered liquorice	40 ,,
Calcium glycerophosphate	1·8 ,,
Extract of gentian	5·0 ,,
Extract of damiana (?)	8 ,,
Alkaloid	0·06 ,,
Water to	100 ,,

In addition, there appeared to be present a slight trace of the oil of one of the umbelliferous fruits, probably anise or fennel. Disregarding the trace of alkaloid, the estimated cost of the ingredients for 1¼ oz. is 2d.

PINK PILLS FOR PALE PEOPLE.

These pills, sold by the Dr. Williams Medicine Company, from an address in London, are stated to be manufactured in the United States of America. The price is 2s. 9d. a box, containing 30 pills.

The pills are advertised for a great variety of diseases, prominence being usually given to one disease in each advertisement; thus four long advertisements appearing simultaneously in different papers were respectively headed:

Afraid of being touched. So sore with Rheumatism. A once-crippled victim tells how Dr. Williams' Pink Pills cleansed his system of Rheumatism.

Eczema expelled. Mr. John Chamberlain tells how his sufferings from Skin Disease were cured by Dr. Williams' Pink Pills.

Sciatica's Swift Pains rendered this Lady helpless. Her case had defied treatment, but Dr. Williams' Pink Pills succeeded by curing the cause of Sciatica.

The Dark Days of Dyspepsia. . . Dr. Williams' Pink Pills go to the very cause of the mischief.

Each advertisement included a long description of a "case," and as a rule a picture was introduced. The following is from the concluding paragraph of the first of these advertisements, and the others ended in a similar way.

THE DR. WILLIAMS' WAY.

When the muscles and nerves are tortured by poisons in the Blood, be the result Rheumatism, Sciatica, or Lumbago, the only way to a cure is to Enrich and Purify the Blood. Dr. Williams' Pink Pills, in this way alone, have cured not only Rheumatism, but Anæmia, Indigestion, Palpitations, Influenza's After-Effects, Eczema, Sciatica, St. Vitus' Dance, Spinal Weakness, the many forms of Nervous Disorders dreaded by men; also the special ailments of women.

The pills were ovoid in shape and coated with sugar, coloured pink; after removal of the coating they had an average weight of 3 grains. Analysis showed them to contain ferrous sulphate, potassium carbonate (these two having reacted more or less completely, and about one-third of the iron having become oxidized to the ferric state), magnesia, powdered liquorice, and sugar. Since it has been stated that these pills contain arsenic, careful search was made for it, but it was not found. The pill is thus merely one of the many variations of Blaud's pill. The quantities of the different ingredients found indicated the following formula:

Exsiccated sulphate of iron	0·75 grain.
Potassium carbonate, anhydrous	0·66 ,,
Magnesia	0·09 ,,
Powdered liquorice	1·4 ,,
Sugar	0·2 ,,
In one pill.	

The estimated cost of the ingredients for 30 pills is one-tenth of a penny.

BEECHAM'S PILLS.

A box of these pills, advertised to be worth a guinea, is sold for 1s. 1½d., and the prime cost of the ingredients of the 56 pills it contains is about half a farthing.

In a circular wrapped round the box it is stated that "these renowned pills are composed entirely of Medicinal Herbs," and cure Constipation, Headache, Dizziness or Swimming in the Head, Wind, Pain, and Spasms at the Stomach, Pains in the Back, Restlessness, Insomnia, Indigestion, Want of Appetite, Fullness after Meals, Vomitings, Sickness of the Stomach, Bilious or Liver Complaints, Sick Headaches, Cold Chills, Flushings of Heat, Lowness of Spirits, and all Nervous Affections, Scurvy and Scorbutic Affections, Pimples and Blotches on the Skin, Bad Legs, Ulcers, Wounds, Maladies of Indiscretion, Kidney and Urinary Disorders, and Menstrual Derangements.

The pills had an average weight of 1¼ grains, and analysis showed them to consist of aloes, ginger, and soap; no other medicinal ingredient was found. The quantities were approximately as follows:

Aloes	0·5 grain.
Powdered ginger	0·55 ,,
Powdered soap	0·18 ,,
In one pill.	

NERVLETTES.

Of these pills, which are sold in a bottle, price 1s. 1½d., containing 27 pills, a circular enclosed in the package said

Coleman's Nervlettes or Nerve Pills generate brain and nerve-force.

The pills were coated with talc; after removal of the coating they had an average weight of about 1½ grains. Analysis showed them to contain free phosphorus, quinine sulphate, a little powdered liquorice, and about 20 per cent. of a powdered vegetable tissue, which could not be identified; the remainder of the pill appeared to be of the nature of excipient only. The amounts of phosphorus and quinine were determined, and indicated the following formula:

Phosphorus	0·005 grain.
Quinine sulphate	0·07 ,,
Vegetable-powder	0·3 ,,
In one pill.	

MOTHER SEIGEL'S CURATIVE SYRUP.

The price of a bottle of Mother Seigel's Syrup containing 3 fluid ounces is 2s. 6d.

Although this was described on the wrapper as "for dyspepsia" so many disorders were stated to be due to this cause, and amenable to treatment with this preparation, that it may fairly be included in this chapter. On the other side of the wrapper it was called "A cure for impurities of the blood," and "A cure for dyspepsia and liver complaints." In a circular enclosed with the bottle it was stated:

The symptoms mentioned above are the smoke of the fire of indigestion—a fire that will eat out your very vitals and sap your strength and vitality. For it can't be too often repeated that indigestion is the root of a great deal of evil; the origin of a great many disorders which no man quite understands how he came by. And why this is can easily be explained. Disease is poison; its symptoms are the manifestation of the poison. Indigestion creates many dangerous poisons, and is therefore the cause of many diseases.

So let us get rid of the smoke by putting out the fire, and purify our blood and system with Mother Seigel's Syrup, which will sweep away the poisons and make us healthy and strong.

Mother Seigel's Syrup is a highly concentrated, purely vegetable compound, having a specific action on the stomach, liver, and kidneys.

Analysis showed the presence of free hydrochloric acid, which is not usually classified as a vegetable compound, tincture of capsicum, a bitter substance agreeing in its properties with aloes, and sugar (partly as invert sugar); the colouring and flavouring substances also present indicated that the sugar had been added in the form of treacle. Quantitative determination of those ingredients capable of it, and estimation of the others by comparison with known mixtures, indicated the following formula:

Dilute hydrochloric acid (*B.P.*)	....	10 parts by measure.
Tincture of capsicum	....	1·7 ,, ,,
Aloes	....	2 parts.
Treacle	....	60 ,,
Water to	....	100 parts by measure.

The estimated cost of the ingredients for 3 fluid ounces is one-third of a penny.

THE ILLS OF HUMANITY.

SEVERAL examples have been encountered in previous chapters of the system of getting into personal communication with a possible customer, and addressing to him a series of letters warning him of the dire consequences should he fail to purchase the advertiser's "treatment." Over and beyond the chance of frightening the customer, the system, which seems to have originated in the United States of America, has the advantages that a profession can be made of adapting the treatment to the individual case, that the price may be lowered if the charge first made is considered too high and that possibly, in return for this concession, testimonials and the names of other sufferers may be obtained. A letter-writing system of this kind is found at work behind the advertisement from which the following paragraphs are extracted:

Free! Free!

To the Sick and Ailing Everywhere.

The Cure for your Disease—Delivered Free—Free for the Asking—Free to You.

To the sick—the suffering—to every man and woman victim of organic disease—local trouble or broken general health—Dr. Kidd's offer of free treatments is given in the absolute faith and sincere belief that they can and will stop disease, cure it, and lift you up again to health and vigour. . .

Rheumatism, kidney trouble, Bright's disease, diabetes, heart disease, partial paralysis, bladder troubles, stomach and bowel troubles, piles, catarrh, bronchitis, weak lungs, consumption, asthma, chronic coughs, nervousness, all female troubles, lumbago, skin diseases, scrofula, impure blood, general debility, organic vital ailments, etc., are cured to remain and continue cured . . . .

Will you let me do this for you—will you let me prove it—brother and sister sufferers? Are you willing to trust a master physician, who not only MAKES this offer, but PUBLISHES it and then sends the test and proof of his remedies without a penny of cost to anyone except himself? . . .

My home office is at Fort Wayne, Indiana. U.S.A., but for the benefit of my thousands of English patients, I have established an office in London. Please address Dr. James W. Kidd, " Box " No. . . . , E.C.

The advertisement was illustrated by the portrait of a man who, it might be assumed, was the " master physician " in question, but that in a book of some hundred pages, entitled " The Ills of Humanity, by Dr. James W. Kidd, Fort Wayne, Ind.," issued apparently by " the J. W. Kidd Co.," there is a portrait of Dr. James W. Kidd, which seems to represent a totally different person.

The book is principally occupied with a series of paragraphs on different complaints, rather over a hundred being dealt with ; in the majority of cases the description leads up to reference to Dr. Kidd's treatment, or medicines, etc. Dr. James William Kidd, the book states, possesses a profound knowledge of medicine, a remarkable power over disease, and has " among his resources remedies that enable him to treat successfully many diseases that are generally considered incurable." After this the fact disclosed by analysis that his remedies seem in reality sadly lacking in originality and novelty, must excite a mild surprise.

It appears that persons writing to Dr. James W. Kidd, or the J. W. Kidd Co., receive a " Self-Examination and Consultation Blank." In one instance in which the blank was filled up, the reply was as follows :

Diagnosis and Case Record.
By Dr. James W. Kidd, Fort Wayne, Ind.

For a complete description of your case, the probable results and my method of treatment, see pages 46, 99, 29, 13, 9, of the pamphlet " The Ills of Humanity," sent you under separate cover.

I find that you are afflicted with Rheumatism, Scrofula, Catarrh, Dyspepsia and Gastritis.

Rheumatism MEANS an excess of uric acid in the blood.

Scrofula is a constitutional disease almost synonymous with tuberculosis.

Catarrh is an excreting inflammation of the mucous membrane.

Dyspepsia (Indigestion) MEANS impaired secretion of pepsin and consequent imperfect digestion.

Gastritis MEANS catarrh of the mucous membrane of the stomach.

TAKE THE REMEDIES ACCORDING TO THE FOLLOWING DIRECTIONS:

One Tablet " A " before breakfast.
One Tablet " B " before dinner.
One Tablet No. 18 before supper.
One Tablet No. 7 after dinner and after supper.
One Tablet No. 45 on retiring.

This was accompanied by tablets marked " A," " B," and " 18," three of each, four marked " 45," and five marked " 7 "; also by a letter which appeared to be lithographed, and although the name and address were in the same writing and the same ink, they showed evidence of having been added afterwards. It seems probable, therefore, that, although professing to be a personal letter, it was one in regular use. It stated that Dr. James W. Kidd has " to-day selected and will forward to your address upon receipt of your remittance of 1l. the complete course of treatment," the tablets sent being only samples. The letter apologizes for the smallness of the samples on the ground that the drugs " are very expensive." The writer adds: " I have taken special interest in your case, because I want a cured patient in your immediate vicinity." The tablets were analysed as completely as was possible with the small quantities sent, with the following results:

Tablet A (triangular) was coloured externally with a salmon-pink dye; the outer coating was of sugar, and below this was a rather thick coating of chalk, forming a very hard and resistant covering to the tablet. The decoated tablets weighed about $3\frac{1}{4}$ grains each; they contained 52 per cent. of sodium bicarbonate, and the remainder consisted principally of a bitter extract agreeing in all respects with extract of gentian; small quantities of potato starch and a substance of resinoid nature, which could not be identified, were also present. No other medicinal substance could be found.

Tablet B (triangular) was coloured externally with a bluish-purple dye; the coating and the material of the tablets agreed in all respects with Tablet A, and the two were apparently identical

Tablet 18 (circular) was white; the coating was of similar composition to that of A. The decoated tablets weighed about 3·8 grains each; analysis showed the presence of about 1 grain of sodium benzoate in each, together with a small quantity of a greenish, moderately bitter resin which could not be identified, and a trace of oil of wintergreen. Faint indications were obtained of a trace of an alkaloid, but not enough to amount to positive evidence. No other medicinal substance could be found; the remainder was of "extractive" nature.

Tablet 45 (circular) was coloured externally with a pink dye; the coating was of similar composition to that of A. The decoated tablets weighed about 1·1 grain each; the chief constituent was aloes, and there was also present a very small quantity of ginger extract, and a small quantity of a resin, which was probably jalap or scammony resin; also a moderate trace of alkaloid, which was not the alkaloid of nux vomica, belladonna, or hyoscyamus, but was not present in quantity sufficient to be identified; the only other ingredient found was a little potato starch.

Tablet 7 (circular) was not coated. The average weight of these was 6·5 grains each, and they consisted principally of charcoal, with some sugar and a very little saccharin.

"These special remedies are very expensive!"

BURGESS'S LION OINTMENT.

The results of an examination of Burgess's Lion Ointment may be given here inasmuch as it will be seen that it is recommended for the cure of a great number of disorders. It is supplied in boxes at 1s. 1½d., 2s. 9d., 4s. 6d., 11s., and jars at 22s.; the 1s. 1½d. box contains 1 oz., and the next size 3 oz.

A circular wrapped round the box was headed "Amputation avoided—the knife superseded," and continued:

> E. Burgess's Lion Ointment and Pills Have deservedly become the popular remedies for curing all diseases of the Skin, Old Wounds, Ulcers, Abscesses, (including Tuberculous), Tumours, Polypuses, Piles, Fistulas, Shingles, Venereal

Sores, Whitlows, Broken Breasts, Bad Legs, Boils, Scurvy, Scrofula (*King's Evil*), Scorbutic Eruptions, Poisoned Wounds *of all kinds*, Stings, Venomous Bites, Scurf, Ringworm, Itch, Corns, Chilblains, Chapped Hands, Cracked Lips, Cuts, Burns, Scalds, Gatherings in the Ear, Toothache, Earache, Neuralgia, Rheumatism, Gout, Sciatica, Quinsey, Bronchitis, Asthma, Deafness, etc.; also Ulcerous Affections of the Womb, for the treatment of which apply to the Proprietor, personally, or by letter, *in all cases free*. These invaluable medicines have not been introduced as remedies for any of the above complaints, or diseases, until they have in each case PRACTICALLY proved EFFECTUAL. To those who are suffering from diseases *apparently* rendering amputation necessary, they are especially recommended, as they entirely do away with the necessity for the same by drawing all the cause of the disease from the affected part, cleansing the blood, and restoring the system to a sound, healthy condition.

They are vegetable preparations, and the Ointment can be applied with perfect confidence to the most tender skin. It is entirely free from all poisonous ingredients, a great recommendation for the nursery—for which it is invaluable.

In spite of the ointment being a "vegetable preparation," analysis showed the principal ingredient to be lead oleate (lead plaster); this is blended with resin, wax, and fatty ingredients; vegetable extracts and active principles were found to be absent. It is not possible to separate the ingredients of an ointment like this sharply one from another; and, since the ingredients are not themselves simple bodies but mixtures liable to rather wide variations, they can only be approximately determined, and, as regards the lard and oil, even identification cannot be placed beyond doubt nor can small quantities of some other fats be certainly stated to be absent. These, however, are matters of minor importance. The composition given below has been checked by varying the analytical methods, as well as by comparison of various ointments prepared according to formulæ suggested by analysis. As a result of the investigation, the following formula was arrived at, which gives an ointment similar to the "Lion" ointment:

Lead-plaster	13 parts.
Beeswax	20 ,,
Resin	11 ,,
Olive oil	12 ,,
Water	6 ,,
Lard, to	100 ,,

The estimated cost of the ingredients is about 10d. per ℔. of ointment.

APPENDIX.

STAMP DUTY ON SECRET REMEDIES.

The duty on secret medicines is regulated by the Stamp Act of 1804 as amended by the Stamp Act Amendment Act of 1812. The Act of 1804 was itself in part an amending Act and regulated the duties to be paid on paper, on books, on advertisements, and imposed *ad valorem* duties on hats and proprietary medicines. The tax on proprietary medicines remains, but that on advertisements through and by which they continue to exist and flourish has gone the way of the duties on hats, and books, and paper. The Act of 1804 contained a schedule of medicines to the number of some 450. In the Act of 1812 this was replaced by a new schedule in which about 550 proprietary medicines were mentioned by name. The final clause of this Act, however, is expressed in very general terms, for it includes "all other pills, powders, lozenges, tinctures, potions, cordials, electuaries, plasters, unguents, salves, ointments, drops, lotions, oils, spirits, medicated herbs and waters, chemical and officinal preparations whatsoever, to be used or applied externally or internally as medicines or medicaments for the prevention, cure, or relief of any disorder or complaint incident to or in any wise affecting the human body," if the person making or selling these various preparations claim to have any occult secret or art for making them, or claim to have any exclusive right or title to make them, or prepares and sells them under the authority of letters patent, or if by public notice or advertisement, or by papers or labels on, or with, the enclosures, bottles, or cases in which the preparation is sold, the maker, vendor, or proprietor recommend them as "nostrums, or as proprietary medicines, or as specifics, or as beneficial to the prevention, cure, or relief of any distemper, malady, ailment, disorder, or complaint incident to or in any wise affecting the human body."

The Inland Revenue returns show that during the last ten years the amount received by the State from the stamp duty on patent medicines so-called has increased from £266,403 10s. 3d. in the year ending March 31, 1899, to £334,141 19s. 2½d. in the year ending March 31st, 1908. The net receipts are the gross receipts after deducting repayments and allowances, but the aggregates of these deductions are small. The following table shows the net receipts in each of the ten years, and the average for the two quinquennial periods, 1899-1903 and 1904-1908 :—

TABLE SHOWING NET RECEIPTS FROM STAMPS ON "PATENT MEDICINES" FOR TEN YEARS, 1899-1908.

Year.	Yearly.	Quinquennial average.
	£ s. d.	£ s. d.
1899	266,403 10 3	
1900	288,827 8 1½	
1901	297,479 19 6	298,483 18 3
1902	306,337 5 9	
1903	333,371 7 9	
1904	323,445 14 0	
1905	331,438 17 6½	
1906	324,111 14 2	328,048 16 0
1907	327,105 15 3½	
1908	334,141 19 2½	

The value of the stamp which the vendor must affix to the bottle or package varies according to the price charged for the medicine, and the returns show the number of articles for which the several rates are paid. The following table gives the amount of the stamp duty on the several prices, the number of articles stamped in the fiscal year 1908, and the amount of the stamp. An attempt has also been made to estimate the total amount paid by the public for the articles stamped :—

TABLE SHOWING RATES OF DUTY, NUMBER OF ARTICLES STAMPED AND APPROXIMATE SUM PAID BY THE PUBLIC IN THE YEAR ENDING MARCH 31ST, 1908.

Price of Article without stamp.	Stamp.	Number of articles stamped.	Price paid by public.
£ s. d.	s. d.		£ s. d.
0 1 0	0 1½	33,037,202	1,858,342 12 0
0 2 6	0 3	7,565,822	1,040,300 10 0
0 4 0	0 6	1,002,549	225,573 10 6
0 10 0	1 0	122,249	67,236 19 0
1 0 0	2 0	18,445	20,289 10 0
1 10 0	3 0	11,308	18,658 4 0
		41,757,575	3,230,401 5 6

This estimate of the total amount paid by the public must be too high. In the first place it will be seen that the stamp duty does not rise by regular increments *ad valorem*. An article, the nominal price of which is 1s., must bear a stamp of 1½d., but if the nominal price be 1s. 6d., the stamp is 3d., and for an article of the nominal price of 2s. 6d. it is the same. In the second place, a large proportion of all the articles, probably the great majority of those at 1s., are sold at a discount, "store prices." In the above table the maximum price for each rate of stamp duty and the full nominal prices are assumed. If a deduction of 25 per cent. is made to meet these sources of error, we have a sum of £2,422,800 19s. 1½d., as an estimate of the amount spent by the public on patent medicine in the financial year ending March 31, 1908.

At one time some of the vendors of nostrums took to inserting in their advertisements phrases intended to suggest that the Inland Revenue stamp upon their packages implied some sort of Government guarantee of the efficacy of the remedy. Though the Inland Revenue authorities do not as a rule display any anxiety with regard to the welfare of the public in the matter of the sale of nostrums, their efforts being confined to the collection of the duty, and the enforcement of the provisions of the Act should any vendor show a disposition to evade them, the stamp in recent years has borne the statement "This stamp implies no Government guarantee." In spite of this vendors still sometimes contrive to convey the suggestion that the stamp conveys some sort of government guarantee; the suggestion looks the more plausible if the vendor has his name or autograph printed on the stamp by the government authorities; this will be done for him if he pays the cost of the die, and by the use of such an endorsement the incautious buyer may be led to assume that the Inland Revenue in some way shares the vendors' responsibility for the genuineness of the article, that is to say for the genuineness of its claims. It has been suggested that the Legislature might go further and require the composition and ingredients of any secret remedy to be stated upon the label, box, or package, and looking to the nature of the facts disclosed by the analyses published in this book, it may well be believed that such publications on the labels would act to a certain extent as a warning to the public, for it would be apparent even to the least instructed that the claims in the vendors' circulars were not quite consonant with the commonplace nature of the ingredients of the mixture, powder, pill, lotion, or ointment.

INDEX.

	PAGE
Absorbit Reducing Paste	87
Absorptive Pile Treatment, Van Vleck's	154
Acetanilide (antifebrin)	2, 5, 6, 37, 38, 39, 40, 41, 58, 165
Acetic acid	16, 78
,, ether	16
Acetyl-salicylic acid	56, 59, 60, 64, 77, 81
Act, Stamp	182
Alcohol	7, 8, 12, 14, 16, 17, 19, 26, 32, 44, 47, 52, 73, 74, 78, 80, 86, 87, 92, 103, 111, 118, 121, 127, 135, 160, 167
Allan's Anti-fat	92
Almond, oil of	35, 135, 138
Aloes	48, 49, 55, 104, 175, 176, 177, 180
Aloin	69, 109, 110, 161
Alum	51, 120
Aluminium oleate	120
,, sulphate	145
Ammoniacum	18
Ammoniated mercury	113, 143, 144
Ammonium bromide	126, 128, 129
,, carbonate	125
,, chloride	19
,, citrate	87
Aniseed, oil of	12, 14
,, powdered	18
,, Powell's Balsam of	14
Antexema	105
Anthylla	104
Anti-cataract Mixture, Pomie's	146
Anti-catarrh, Birley's	7
Anticelta Tablets	163
Anti-corpulent Preparation, Russell's	87

	PAGE
Antidipso	165
Anti-epileptic Medicine, W. and J. Taylor's	126
Antiépileptique (Uten)	129
Anti-fat, Allan's	92
Antifebrin (see Acetanilide).	
Antigout soap	64
Antimony oxide	132
Antipon	86
Anti-rheumatic Pearls, Baring Gould's	55
Appendix	182
Aspirin (see Acetyl-salicylic acid).	
Assmann's Whooping Cough Remedy	19
Atropine	163
Augenwol	146
"Bacillentod" (G. Pohl's Family Tea)	36
Baldness, Medicines for (internal)	114
Capsulated Haemoglobin Ovals	115
Capsuloids	114
Haemoglobin Capsules	116
Balsam of Peru	27, 113, 115
Balsamic Cough Mixture, Crosby's	15
Balsamic Elixir, Congreve's	26
Baring Gould's Anti-rheumatic Pearls	55
Barium sulphate	122
Beans, Bile	77
Bearberry (Uvae ursi)	104

	PAGE
Beecham's Cough Pills	18
„ Pills	175
Beeswax 58, 88, 120, 140, 143, 149, 151, 181	
Bell's Fairy Cure	39
Benzoate, Sodium	180
Benzoin, compound tincture of	15, 27
Berberine	80
Berendorf's Powder for Epilepsy	129
Betony	63
Bile Beans	77
Birley's Anti-catarrh	7
Bishop's Gout Varalettes	62
Bladderwrack 83, 84, 89, 91, 92, 93, 94, 100, 102, 103, 104	
Blair's Gout and Rheumatic Pills	50
Blood Cure, Munyon's	44
„ Mixture, Clarke's	42
„ Pills, Harvey's	44
„ „ Hughes's	48
Blood Purifiers	42
Clarke's World-Famed Mixture	42
Harvey's Pills	44
Hood's Compound Extract of Sarsaparilla	46
Hughes's Pills	48
Munyon's Cure	44
Phelps Brown's Purifier	46
Steven's Consumption Cure	21, 28
Townsend's American Sarsaparilla	43
Blue dye	118, 119
Borax	7, 129, 138
Boric acid	106, 109, 113
Bostock's Eye Ointment	143
Brixa Tablets	163
Bromide .... ·	2, 35, 124, 129
„ in Tuberculozyne	35
Brompton Consumption and Cough Specific	27
Brown's Vervain Restorative Assimilant, O. Phelps	127
Bryony	63
Buckthorn	104
Buer's Mul'la	149

	PAGE
Buer's Piles Cure	149
Burdock	45
Burgess's Lion Ointment	180
Caffein	38, 39
Calcium carbonate	6, 109
„ glycerophosphate	173
„ phosphate	132
„ sulphate	28, 109
Calling in the doctor	9, 12
Calomel	113, 131, 132, 148, 151
Camomile	63
Camphor	2, 5, 65, 135, 173
Cancer remedies	117
Cardigan Cancer Curers	121
Caustics and Cancer	122
Canexia preparations	163
Capsicum 14, 35, 69, 156, 160, 176, 177	
Capsulated Haemoglobin Ovals	115
Capsuloids	114
Carbolic acid (see Phenol).	
Cardigan Cancer Curers	121
Carmine	88
Cascara	2, 6, 55, 74, 104, 156, 161
Cascarilla	70
Cassia, oil of	35
Catarrh Balm, Van Vleck's	3
Catarrh Cures	1
Birley's	7
Lane's	2
Munyon's	6
Van Vleck's	3
Catarrh and Cold Cures	1
Birley's	7
Keene's " One Night "	5
Lane's	2
Mackenzie's " One Day "	4
Munyon's	6
Van Vleck's	3
Caulophyllin	80
Caustics and cancer	122
C.B.Q. Tablets, Post's	61
" Century Thermal " Bath Cabinet	99
Charcoal	172
" Chijitse "	22, 32
Children's Cooling Powders, Fenning's	133

	PAGE
Chiretta	168
Chloroform	12, 13, 14, 16, 17, 74, 125
,, spirits of	43
Chlorophyll	111, 112
Cimicifuga	57
Cinchonine	2, 5, 6, 167
Cinnamon, powdered	164
Citric Acid	64, 81, 84, 86, 87
Clarke's Blood Mixture	42
Clifton's Treatment for Deafness	136
Cochineal	27, 35, 86, 120
Cocoa	41
Cocoa-butter (see Theobroma, oil of).	
Cod Liver Oil, Pastor Felke's Honey	36
Colchicin	61, 64
Colchicum	51, 63
Cold Cures	1
Keene's " One Night "	5
Mackenzie's " One Day "	4
Colds in the head	1
Coleman's Nervlettes	175
Collie's Ointment	57
Colza	88, 135
Congreve's Balsamic Elixir	26
Consumption Cures	20
"Bacillentod" (Pohl's Family Tea)	36
Brompton specific	27
Congreve's Balsamic Elixir	26
Felke's Honey Cod Liver Oil, Pastor	36
Kefyr Ferment	24
Körber's	36
Lieber's Tea	36
Pohl's Family Tea (" Bacillentod ")	36
Star Tonic	23
Steven's (Sacco or Lungsava)	21, 28
Tuberculozyne	21, 32
Weidhaas Hygienic Institute	23
Consumption, Körber's Cure for	36
Consumption and Cough specific, Brompton	27

	PAGE
Cooling Powders for Infants	130
Fenning's Children's Powders	133
Pritchard's Teething and Fever Powders	132
Copper in Tuberculozyne	35
,, oleate	120
Corpulence (see Obesity Cures).	
Corpulin	104
Cough Cure, Kilmer's Indian	15
,, ,, Veno's Lightning	16
,, Drops, Lauser's	19
,, ,, Reichel's	19
,, Lozenges, Keating's	17
Cough Medicines	9
Assmann's Whooping Cough Remedy	19
Beecham's Cough Pills	18
Crosby's Balsamic Elixir	15
Kay's Linseed Compound	12
Keating's Lozenges	17
Kilmer's Indian Cure	15
Lauser's Drops	19
Owbridge's Lung Tonic	13
Powell's Balsam of Aniseed	14
Reichel's Drops	19
Tussothym	19
Veno's Lightning Cure	16
Cough Medicines, Morphine in	9, 13, 15, 18, 28
,, ,, Opium in	10, 11, 28
,, Pills, Beecham's	18
,, Specific, Brompton	27
Coza Powder	162
Creasote	113, 152
Crompton's Specific for Deafness	135
Crosby's Balsamic Cough Elixir	15
Cummin, powdered	164
Curative Syrup, Mother Seigel's	176
Cure Alls	170
Beecham's Pills	175
Martin's Miracletts	163
Nervlettes	175
Seigel's Curative Syrup, Mother	176
Therapion	172
Williams' Pink Pills for Pale People	170, 174

Curic Wafers	38
Cuticura remedies	110
Cystamin (*see* Formamine).	
Cystogen (*see* Formamine).	
Daisy Powders	38
Dalloff's Tea	104
Damiana, extract of	173
Daturine	168
Deafness, remedies for ear disease and	134
Clifton's Treatment	136
Crompton's Specific	135
Dellar's Essence	135
Nazaseptic	139
Ohraseptic	139
Ohrsorb Compound	133
Dellar's Essence for Deafness	135
Diabetes Cures	76
A Lancashire nostrum	80
Dill's Mixture	76, 77, 79
Pesqui's Uranium Wine (Vin Urané Pesqui)	76, 77
Diabetic foods	81
,, Mixture, Dill's	76, 77, 79
Dill's Diabetic Mixture	76, 77, 79
Dipsocure	164
Doan's Backache Kidney Pills	67
,, Pile Ointment	151
Dodd's Kidney Pills	69
Drug Cures for Inebriety	168
Duboisine	168
Duty on Secret Remedies, Stamp	182
Ear disease (*see* Deafness, Remedies for).	
Ekzemin Cream	113
Electricum	64
Eosin	91
Epilepsy, Remedies for	124
Antiépileptique (Uten)	129
Berendorf's Powder	129
Lamma Powder	129
Osborne's Mixture	126
Ozerine	125
Phelps Brown's Vervain Restorative Assimilant	127

Epilepsy, Remedies for—contd.—	
Taylor's Anti-epileptic Medicine, W. and J.	126
Trench's Remedy	127
Essence for Deafness, Dellar's	135
Eucalyptus	4, 112
Eye diseases, Remedies for	142
Augenwol	146
Bostock's Ointment	143
"New and Marvellous Remedy"	144
Okterin	146
Opthalmol	146
Pomie's Anticataract Mixture	146
Singleton's Ointment	142
Wisbech Remedy	144
Eye Ointment, Bostock's	143
,, Singleton's	142
Fairy Cure, Bell's	39
Felke's Honey Cod Liver Oil, Pastor	36
Fell Reducing Treatment	97
Fenning's Children's Cooling Powders	133
Fenugreek	68
Ferric chloride	121
,, oxide	5, 40, 54, 172
Ferrous sulphate	174
Fever Powders, Pritchard's Teething and	132
Figuroids	94
Fitch's Kidney and Liver Cooler	71
Fits, Trench's Remedy for Epilepsy and	127
Fluorescein	70
Formaldehyde	129
Formamine	85, 96
Fucus vesiculosus (*see* Bladderwrack).	
Galeopsidis	36
Gall stones	79
Galls, powdered	156

	PAGE
Gaultheria, oil of	73
Gelsemium	60
Genoform Tablets	60
Gentian.... 62, 63, 161, 173, 179	
Germicides	31
Ginger 49, 88, 89, 109, 110, 175, 180	
Gloria Tonic	53
Gloria Treatment for Rheumatism	52
Gluten flour	81, 82
Glycerine 17, 30, 32, 35, 73, 74, 78, 89, 90, 92, 93, 103, 113, 120, 135, 138, 142, 143, 144, 146, 173	
Glycerophosphate, calcium	173
Gout, Rheumatism, and Neuralgia, remedies for	50
Baring Gould's Pearls	55
Bishop's Varalettes....	62
Blair's Pills	50
Collie's Ointment	57
Electricum	64
Genoform Tablets	60
Gloria Treatment	52
Gower's Green Pills....	56
Hamm's Cure	51
Laville's Remedies	64
Lazarus Soap	64
Oquit....	59
Pistoia Powders	62
Portland Powder	62
Post's C.B.Q. Tablets	61
Rheuma Tabakolin....	65
Rheumacid	64
Uricedin	64
Weigand's Spirit	65
Zox	58
Gout and Rheumatic Pills, Blair's	50
Gout and Sciatica Cure, Hamm's Rheumatic	51
Gout Powders, Pistoia	62
,, ,, Portland	62
,, Varalettes, Bishop's	62
Gower's Green Pills	56
Graziana Reducing Treatment (Zehrkur)	103
Green Pills, Gower's	56
Grindelia robusta	17

	PAGE
Guaiacum	44, 54, 62, 64
Guarantee bonds	30
Haemoglobin	114, 115, 116
,, Capsules	116
,, Ovals, Capsulated	115
Haemorrhoids (*see* Piles, Remedies for).	
Hair (*see* Baldness).	
Hamamelidis	150
Hamamelin	152
Hamamelis (witch hazel) 148, 149, 152	
Hamm's Rheumatic, Gout, and Sciatica Cure	51
Hargreave's Reducing Wafers	91
Harmless Headache Powders, Hoffman's	41
Harvey's Blood Pills	44
Headache	37
,, Cure, Stearns's	39
Headache Powders	37
Bell's Fairy Cure	39
Curic Wafers	38
Daisy....	38
" Good as Gold "	41
Hoffman's Harmless	41
Kaputine	40
Retailers supplying....	41
Stearns's Cure	39
Healine Treatment for Rupture	160
Hemlock pitch....	68
Hemotora	153
Henbane	69, 71
Hexamethylene-tetramine (*see* Formamine).	
Hoffman's Harmless Headache Powders	41
Homatropine	168, 169
Hood's Compound Extract of Sarsaparilla	46
Hughes's Blood Pills	48
Hydrastine	80
Hydrastis	77, 80
Hydrochloric acid	121, 169, 176, 177
Hyoscine	168, 169
Hyoscyamine	168, 169

	PAGE
Icthyol	140, 151
Ills of humanity	177
Burgess's Lion Ointment	180
Kidd's Treatment	178
Indian Cough Cure, Kilmer's....	15
Inebriety, cures for	162
Antidipso	165
Coza Powder	162
Dipsocure	164
Drug cures, some other	168
Teetolia Treatment....	166
Inebriety, drug cures for	168
Iodine 84, 94, 102, 103,	126
,, tincture....	126
Ipecacuanha 2, 11, 12, 13, 14, 18, 28	
Iridin	157
Iron 71, 87, 89, 121,	162
,, chloride	121
,, phosphate	89
,, sulphate	175
Jalap 48, 49, 55, 57, 69, 70,	180
Jaundice	72, 79
Juniper.... .... 66, 68,	71
,, preparations	113
J.Z. Obesity Tablets	87
Kaolin 54, 109,	172
Kaputine	40
Kay's Linseed Compound	12
,, Linum Catharticum Pills	12
Keating's Cough Lozenges	17
Keene's "One Night" Cold Cure	5
Kefyr	23
Kidd's Treatment, James W.....	178
Kidney medicines	66
Doan's Pills	67
Dodd's Pills	69
Fitch's Kidney and Liver Cooler	71
Munyon's Cure	75
Var's American Pills	70
Veno's Seaweed Tonic	74
Warner's Cure	72
Kidney Pills, Doan's Backache	67

	PAGE
Kilmer's Indian Cough Cure	15
Kino	32
Körber's Cure for Consumption	36
Krameria, decoction of	32
Kupfinn, "Dr."	139
Lactose (*see* Milk sugar).	
Lamma Powder	129
Lancashire Nostrum, A	80
Lane's Catarrh Cure	2
Lanoline 149,	154
Lauser's Cough Drops....	19
Lavender	104
Laville's Antigout remedies	64
Laxatol (*see* Phenolphthalein).	
Laxen (*see* Phenolphthalein).	
Laxoin (*see* Phenolphthalein).	
Lazarus Gout and Rheumatic Soap	64
Lead	122
,, acetate 113, 127, 148,	152
,, oleate 113, 119,	181
,, oxide (litharge) 143,	144
,, plaster	181
,, sub-acetate	127
Lemon	84
,, grass	113
,, oil	65
Leptandrin	74
Lieber's Tea for Consumption	36
Lime-juice	77, 81
Linseed compound, Kay's	12
Lion Ointment, Burgess's	180
Liquorice 11, 14, 18, 19, 45, 54, 55, 61, 69, 89, 91, 102, 103, 133, 156, 173, 174, 175, 176	
Lithium citrate	62
Liver Cooler, Fitch's Kidney and	71
LLoyd Reducing Treatment, Nelson	100
Lotion, X.L. Reducing Pills and	89
Lungsava	28
Lung Tonic, Owbridge's	13
Lycopodium	71
Lymphol, Rice's	158

	PAGE
Mackenzie's "One Day" Cold Cure	4
Magnesia	61, 109, 119, 174, 175
„ calcined	150
Magnesium	71, 91, 119
Malachite green	111
Mandelyl-tropeine (see Homatropine).	
Marmola	85, 93
Martin's Miracletts	171
Medicine Stamp Act	182
Medi-cone Pile Treatment, Oxien	151
Menthol	156, 172
Mercuric oxide	143
Mercury, ammoniated	113, 143, 144
Methyl, orange	86
Metramine (see Formamine).	
Milk sugar (lactose)	19, 39, 56, 100, 131, 132, 165, 166
Miracletts, Martin's	171
Mixture for Epilepsy, Osbornes'	126
Mother Seigel's Curative Syrup	176
Muco-Food Cones (Van Vleck's)	148, 155
Mul'la, Buer's	149
Munyon's Catarrh Tablets	6
„ Catarrh Cure	6
„ Blood Cure	44
„ Kidney Cure	75
„ Pile Ointment	150
Nazaseptic	139
Nelson Lloyd Reducing Treatment	100
Nerve stimulators	31
Nervlettes, Coleman's	175
Nettle	36
Neuralgia (see Gout, Rheumatism and Neuralgia, remedies for).	
"New and Marvellous Remedy for the Eyes"	144
Nitre (see Potassium nitrate).	
"No cure no pay"	5, 29, 95
Nostrum, A Lancashire	80

	PAGE
Obesity cures	83
Absorbit Paste and J. Z. Tablets (Zobiede)	87
Allan's Anti-fat	92
Anticelta Tablets	163
Antipon	86
Corpulin and Dalloff's Tea	104
Dalloff's Tea and Corpulin	104
Fell Treatment	97
Figuroids	94
Graziana Treatment (Zehrkur)	103
Hargreave's Wafers	91
J. Z. Tablets and Absorbit Paste	87
Marmola	85, 93
Nelson LLoyd Treatment	100
Russell's Anti-corpulent Preparation	87
Trilene Tablets	90
X.L. Pills and Lotion	89
Zehrkur (Graziana Treatment)	103
Zobiede (Absorbit Paste and J. Z. Tablets)	87
Obesity Tablets, J. Z.	87
Ohraseptic	139
Ohrsorb Compound	138
Oil, Pastor Felke's Honey Cod Liver	36
Ointment, Collie's	57
Okterin	146
Oleic acid	115, 161
Opthalmol	146
Oquit	59
Origanum, oil of (see Thyme).	
Osborne's Mixture for Epilepsy	126
Owbridge's Lung Tonic	13
Ox-bile	88
Oxien Medi-cone Pile Treatment	151
Ozerine	125
Paciderma Blood Wafers	109
„ cream	109
„ powder	109
„ preparations	106

	PAGE
Pale People, Williams' Pink Pills for	170, 174
Paraffin....	4, 70, 100, 106, 109, 110, 111, 112, 113, 120, 140, 143, 144, 146, 151, 152, 156
Patients' names, obtaining	25
Peppermint	14, 36, 69, 71, 77, 81, 94, 127, 160
Pepsin	76
Pesqui's Uranium Wine	76, 77
Petroleum jelly	58, 156
Phelps Brown's Blood Purifier	46
„ „ Vervain Restorative Assimilant....	127
Phenacetin	38, 39
Phenol (carbolic acid)....	1, 3, 4, 7, 120, 151
Phenolphthalein	77, 81, 85, 94, 96, 97
Pheun Skin Paste	113
Phosphoric acid	8
Phosphorus	176
Phytolaccin	54
Pile Ointment, Doan's	151
„ Munyon's	150
Piles, remedies for	147
Buer's Cure	149
„ Mul'la	149
Doan's Ointment	151
Hemotora	153
Muco - food cones (Van Vleck's)	148
Munyon's Ointment	150
Oxien Medi-cone Treatment	151
Rollo's Remedy	153
Van Vleck's Absorptive Treatment	154
Pills, Kay's Linum Catharticum	12
Pine preparations	64
Piperazine	62
Pistoia Gout Powders....	62
Plasma, Van Vleck's	155
Podophyllin	69
Pohl's Family Tea ("Bacillentod")	36
Pomies Anti-cataract Mixture	146
Portland Gout Powder	62
Post's C.B.Q. Tablets	61

	PAGE
Potassium bromide	89, 90, 125, 126, 127, 128, 129, 165, 166
„ carbonate	174, 175
„ chlorate	133
„ chloride	89, 90, 125
„ iodide	43, 45, 47, 52, 54, 61, 89, 90, 92, 93, 111, 126, 142, 146
„ nitrate	66, 68, 70, 71, 72, 73
Powders, headache	37
Daisy	38
"Good as Gold"	41
Hoffman's Harmless	41
Powell's Balsam of Aniseed	14
Prescriptions, secret remedies said to be made from physicians'	27, 38, 59, 80, 108
Pritchard's Teething and Fever Powders	132
Pumilio pine	4, 15
Purgen (*see* Phenolphthalein).	
Quinine	2, 45, 61, 64, 167
„ sulphate	176
„ valerianate	172
Rapeseed (*see* Colza).	
Reducing Paste, Absorbit	87
„ Pills and Lotion, X.L.	89
„ Treatment, Fell	97
„ „ Graziana (Zehrkur)	103
Reducing Treatment, Nelson Lloyd	100
Reducing Wafers, Hargreave's	91
Reichel's Cough Drops	19
Resin, black	58
„ (colophony)	58, 112
„ plasters	119
Retailers, headache powders supplied by	41
Rheuma Tabakolin	65
Rheumacid	64
Rheumatic, Gout, and Sciatica Cure, Hamm's	51

	PAGE
Rheumatic and Gout Spirit, Weigand's	65
Rheumatic Pills, Blair's Gout and	50
Rheumatism (see Gout, Rheumatism, and Neuralgia, remedies for).	
Rheumatism, Gloria Treatment for	52
Rhubarb 45, 55, 74, 104, 111	
Rice's Lymphol	158
,, Treatment for Rupture	158
Rino Ointment....	113
Rock Rose	46
Rollo's Remedy for Piles	153
Rupture, preparations for	158
Healine Treatment	160
Rice's Treatment	158
Russell's Anti-corpulent Preparation	87
Saccharin 11, 172	
Sacco	28
Salicylate, alkaline	57
,, sodium	52
Salicylic acid 92, 93, 113	
,, Methylene-glycol-ester of	61
Saltpetre (see Potassium nitrate).	
Sal volatile	43
Sarsaparilla, compound solution of	44
Sarsaparilla, Hood's Extract of	46
,, Townsend's American	43
Sassafras, oil of	44
Scammony 80, 180	
Sciatica (see Gout, Rheumatism and Neuralgia, remedies for).	
Sciatica Cure, Hamm's Rheumatic, Gout, and	51
Scopolamine	168
Seaweed Tonic, Veno's	74
Seigel's Curative Syrup, Mother	176
Senna 19, 74, 104	

	PAGE
Singleton's Eye Ointment	142
Skin diseases, cures for	105
Antexema	105
Cuticura Remedies	110
Ekzemin Cream	113
Juniper preparations	118
Paciderma preparations	106
Pheun Skin Paste	113
Rino Ointment	113
Zam-buk	111
Zip Ointment	112
Skin Paste, Pheun	113
Soap 57, 64, 65, 70, 113, 119, 135, 140, 175	
,, Antigout....	64
,, Lazarus Gout and Rheumatic	64
Soda alum 142, 145	
Sodium benzoate (see Benzoate).	
Sodium bicarbonate 7, 41, 62, 70, 80, 96, 97, 109, 164, 179	
,, bromide	129
,, chloride 1, 3, 7, 94, 96, 97, 146	
,, phosphate	74
,, sulphate 77, 81, 120, 145	
Soothing powders for infants....	130
Steedman's Powders	131
Soothing, teething and cooling powders for infants	130
Fenning's Children's Powders	133
Pritchard's Powders	132
Stedman's Powders....	130
Steedman's Powders	131
Spearmint	160
Specific for Deafness, Crompton's	135
Spirit, Weigand's Rheumatic and Gout	65
Stamp Act	182
,, on secret remedies	182
Star Tonic	23
Stearns's Headache Cure	39
Stedman's Teething Powders	130
Steedman's Soothing Powders	131
Steven's Consumption Cure 21, 28	
Stillingia	46

	PAGE
Storax	27, 115
"Stramonine"	168
Sulphur	88, 140
„ precipitated	109, 113, 150
Sulphuric acid	16
Tabakolin, Rheuma	65
Tablets, Munyon's Catarrh	6
„ Trilene	90
Talc	5, 54, 57, 59, 96, 97, 109, 156, 161, 172, 176
Tannin	27, 32, 73, 152, 153, 161
Tar	119
Taraxacum	45, 66, 71, 73
Tartaric acid	8, 62, 78, 96, 97
Taylor's anti-epileptic medicine, W. and J.	126
Tea, Dalloff's "Contre l'Obesité"	104
Tea, Lieber's (for Consumption)	36
„ Pohl's Family ("Bacillentod")	36
Teething powders for infants	130
Pritchard's Teething and Fever Powders	132
Stedman's Powders	130
Teetolia Treatment	166
Terebene	118, 119
Theobroma, oil of (cocoa-butter)	148, 152, 154, 156
Therapion	172
Thermal Bath Cabinet "Century"	99
Thyme (oil of Origanum)	19, 160
Thyroid Extract	84, 94, 102, 103
Tolu	13, 16, 18, 27
Tonic, Gloria	52
„ Owbridge's Lung	13
„ Star	23
„ Veno's Seaweed	74
„ Zox	58
Townsend's American Sarsaparilla	43
Tragacanth	106
Trench's Remedy for Epilepsy and Fits	127
Trilene Tablets	90

	PAGE
Tropyltropeine (see Atropine).	
Tuberculozyne	21, 32
Tumenol	140
Turmeric	70
Turpentine	65, 113, 122, 136
Tussothym	19
"Umckaloabo"	22, 32
Uranium nitrate	76, 78, 79
„ Wine, Pesqui's	76, 77
Uricedin	64
Urisol (see Formamine).	
Urotropine (see Formamine).	
Valerianate, Quinine, Zinc	172
Van Vleck's Absorptive Pile Treatment	154
Van Vleck's Catarrh Balm	3
„ „ Muco-food Cones (Pile Treatment)	143
Van Vleck's Pile Pills	155
„ „ Plasma (Pile Treatment)	155
Var's American Kidney Pills	70
Varalettes, Bishop's, Gout	62
Varicocele	161
Varicose veins	161
Veno's Lightning Cough Cure	16
„ Seaweed Tonic	74
Verbena officinalis (see Vervain).	
Vervain Restorative Assimilant, O. Phelps Brown's	127
Vervain (*Verbena officinalis*)	124, 125, 127
Vesalvine (see Formamine).	
Vin Urané Pesqui	76, 77
Wafers, Curic	38
„ Hargreave's Reducing	91
„ Paciderma Blood	109
Warner's Cure	72
Weidhaas Hygienic Institute	23
Weigand's Rheumatic and Gout Spirit	65

	PAGE
White precipitate (*see* Ammoniated mercury).	
Whooping Cough Remedy, Assmann's	19
Williams' Pink Pills for Pale People	170, 174
Wine, Pesqui's Uranium	76, 77
,, spirit of....	32
Wintergreen, oil of	73, 180
Wisbech Remedy for the Eyes	144
Witch hazel (*see* Hamamelis).	
Xaxa (*see* Acetyl-salicylic acid)	
X.L. Reducing Pills and Lotion	89

	PAGE
Yonkerman Company (Tuberculozyne)	32
Zam-buk	111
Zehrkur (*see* Graziana Reducing Treatment)....	103
Zinc	156
,, chloride	122
,, oxide	109, 129, 148, 151
,, sulphate	120
,, valerianate	172
Zip Ointment	112
Zobeida (*see* Zobeide).	
Zobeide	87
Zox	58

PRINTED BY
BRITISH MEDICAL ASSOCIATION,
429, STRAND, LONDON.

Lightning Source UK Ltd.
Milton Keynes UK
UKHW01f1113110918
328700UK00006B/894/P